# Contents

# Acknowledgments

Taking care of a patient in an emergency room or shepherding a bill through the legislative process—both are cooperative endeavors, impossible to achieve by oneself. I've learned that writing a book also requires many helping hands.

Foremost among them is Shelley Cole Morhaim, my life's partner for 36 years, and in many ways the coauthor of this book. She labored with me over every idea, every draft, and every word. This book would not exist without her.

I'm grateful to all the patients who entrusted me with their care. It is a privilege to be able to help people dealing with everything from the most minor conditions to life-threatening illness and injury. They have taught me so much.

*The Better End* began with a research project that evolved from my work at the Johns Hopkins Bloomberg School of Public Health and became a reality due to the hard work and talent of Dr. Keshia Pollack and the support of Dr. Clarence Lam, Dr. Michael Williams, Dr. Ellen Mackenzie, Dr. Michael Klag, Dr. Shannon Frattaroli, Michael Merson, and Bill Casey. In both her life and death, my colleague and sister-in-law, Mary Lou Cole, was a help and inspiration.

My colleagues in the Maryland General Assembly have helped to shape my understanding of how government can best empower citizens to take control of what is a deeply private right. My constituents in Maryland's 11th District have honored me with their trust and guided me with their advice. It's impossible for any legislator to be an expert on all the issues that come before him or her. The public doesn't always realize how much we depend on their input.

I'm grateful to my medical colleagues, and especially to Dr. Michael Auerbach, an unfailing source of wisdom and support.

At key moments in the writing of this book, I've had help from my daughters, Emily, Sarah, and Elizabeth, and from my friends Jan Houbolt, Mike Reed, Jim Kunz, David Heath, Andy Gruver, David Kandel, Brent Flickinger, Geoff Basik, Bob Brown, George Kosmides, Margie von Rueden, Ben Pomerantz, Bonnie Pastor, and Susan Sarno.

I'm also grateful to Bob Silverstein of Quicksilver Books and to Jackie Wehmueller of the Johns Hopkins University Press for believing in the work of a first-time author. Jackie offered cogent advice and critiques all along the way. It's been a pleasure and an education to work with an editor who knows her craft so well.

# The Better End

# Introduction

## Then and Now

Let's go back in time 100 years.

At age 50, Harold Johnson, a farmer in western Pennsylvania, had already exceeded the average life expectancy for his era. Two of his siblings and one of his own children had passed away before reaching the age of 20. A daughter-in-law had died in childbirth. Despite these losses, Harold had enjoyed a full life with Martha, his wife of 26 years, with whom he had four living children and two grandchildren.

But now Harold's life was nearing its close. He developed a bad cold that lingered over the winter. It seemed to intensify the pains he occasionally felt in his chest after physical labor, and he'd had to ask his sons to manage the spring planting without his help. As summer wore on, even the least exertion left him out of breath, until finally he lacked the strength to get out of bed most days.

Dr. Reed, the Johnson family's physician, had trained at Yale Medical College in Connecticut and kept up with all the latest advances. He'd managed to buy Harold a few years of pain relief using nitroglycerin tablets, but as Harold's heart muscle deteriorated, his blood flow decreased. His skin became pale, and fluid began to build up in his lungs, making his breathing even harder. Then pneumonia set in.

When Dr. Reed was called, he confirmed what Harold and Martha suspected: the end was drawing near for Harold. Dr. Reed's scientific medical bag was fairly empty. The antibiotics that could have cured Harold's pneumonia wouldn't be available for another three decades. The cardiac surgery, appliances, and medications that could have repaired his heart's function were even more distantly removed—70 to 90 years in the future. But Dr. Reed wasn't entirely helpless. He'd known the Johnson family for years, and just his presence provided a degree of comfort and dignity to Harold's dying process. Dr. Reed made daily house calls, feeling Harold's pulse, charting the course of his fever and other symptoms, and counseling Harold and Martha. He let them know when it was time to summon the children and grandchildren, the minister from their church, and Harold's brother from Baltimore.

Pneumonia used to be known as "the old person's friend," because it brought a gradual but relatively quick and painless end. As Harold failed, his family and friends came to say goodbye. They talked with Harold about his life and times, both the good and the bad.

As the days progressed, Harold's breathing became more labored, then shallower. He drifted in and out of consciousness. Finally, he lapsed into a coma. With Martha at his side, and his children and grandchildren surrounding his bed, Harold breathed his last.

Now, fast-forward 100 years.

At 83, Harold's great-grandson Bill had already outlived his ancestor by 30-plus years. His three children and five grandchildren all survived into adulthood, and he was able to welcome his first great-grandchild. Bill and his wife, Alice, lived an active life in their community until Bill was diagnosed with prostate cancer at age 75. Surgery and chemotherapy kept the cancer in remission for a number of years, but eventually it returned; this time it did not respond to treatment. As the cancer spread through his body, Bill followed the advice of his oncologist, radiologist, surgeon, and internist. All of them were highly trained specialists and were well versed in the course of Bill's disease, but none knew Bill or Alice very well as individuals.

When Bill's condition moved beyond the help of surgery, his surgeon dropped out of the medical team. When chemotherapy and radiation were no longer options, the specialists in those areas also signed off of Bill's case. His internist prescribed painkillers and made sure the disease was tracked with all appropriate tests, but as Bill's condition worsened, he was moved into the hospital, where his care was largely managed by in-house staff physicians who were strangers to Bill and his family.

Bill underwent multiple hospitalizations over the last 18 months of his life. His children and grandchildren paid visits, but the machinery and organization of the modern medical establishment that kept Bill alive those extra months also served to erect a wall between Bill and his family.

The same type of pneumonia that took his grandfather brought on Bill's final hospitalization. With modern antibiotics, the pneumonia was quickly defeated, leaving Bill's heart to give out after his liver stopped functioning. But instead of dying surrounded by loved ones at his home, he died alone in his cubicle in the intensive care unit (ICU), surrounded by monitors, machines, and intravenous lines, his lungs inflated by a respirator. Since no one felt comfortable declaring the end to be imminent, Alice had gone home for the night, physically exhausted and emotionally drained by the hospital deathwatch.

## Why Not the Best of Both Worlds?

It's not hard to see what's wrong and what's right in each of these scenarios. In the first, Harold gets the benefit of personalized, humane care, with family and friends nearby, but he lacks the life-saving advantages of modern medicine. In the second, thanks to medical advances, Bill enjoys a longer, healthier life, but in his final illness he exchanges the human touch for a succession of specialists, lab tests, x-rays, and hospitalizations. The whole person is reduced to a collection of failing organs and therapies, and he dies isolated from his family and community.

Why can't we have the best of both these worlds? We are the first generation in human history that can actively participate in not only our own health and well-being, but also in our experience of death and dying.

Of course, this won't be true for all of us. Some will die from a sudden lethal stroke or coronary blockage, and others from accidents or other trauma, but the overwhelming majority will succumb to illnesses that once were quickly fatal but are now treatable: cancer, heart ailments, and degenerative diseases. And for most of us, while the exact moment of death is uncertain, generally we can begin to define its circumstances.

Today as we face the end of life, we have a much better sense of what is happening and why. We can approach death with a greater degree of consciousness and information than any of the billions of humans who preceded us. This gives us unprecedented control of how, when, and where we die. Instead of being constrained entirely by the forces of nature, there is now a degree of self-determination in approaching our final passage.

To some extent, this new encounter with the dying process mirrors changes in how we deal with that other universal human experience: childbirth. As medical science developed and had more to offer, childbirth, too, saw an evolution: from attendance by midwives at home to high-tech hospital deliveries managed by trained obstetrical surgeons. Infants and mothers were saved who would have died in former times, but the experience had become isolating for the mother and her family. The requirements of scientific efficiency came to dominate the spiritual and emotional values of simple human connection. But over the past few decades, parents and some medical professionals have demanded changes that re-humanize the process without sacrificing any health benefits. We now see fathers and significant others included in the delivery room. Many hospitals provide homelike birthing centers and support for the laboring mother in the form of nurse-midwives, birth coaches, and prenatal classes for both parents. This evolution is still under way, but it began and continues because ordinary people demanded the "best of both worlds."

Now, as the baby boom generation reaches its senior years, as new lifesaving medical treatments are announced almost weekly, and as our health care system confronts a crisis of affordability, the need is urgent for ordinary people to demand participation in end-of-life decisions. The best, the easiest, and the least expensive way to do this is to complete a form called an "Advance Directive," which allows you to specify the kind of care you want.

## Why This Book?

This book is my attempt to set forth the possible choices that we and our loved ones will face in the course of the dying process. It examines both the medical and legal realities, as well as the options available for decision making. While there is probably no more difficult topic to contemplate than one's own death, there is also the inescapable fact that each of us will die. By thinking about this information now, we can more confidently ensure that our most deeply held values are reflected in the choices made by us or for us during the end-of-life process.

The middle of a health care crisis is the worst time to make difficult or complex decisions, yet it is often exactly when we are called on to do so. The emotional impact of a medical crisis shouldn't be underestimated. Serious illness—whether one's own or that of a spouse, close friend, or family member—is a recognized source of acute stress. During these times our judgment can become clouded, no matter how levelheaded or stoic we may normally be. Complex medical, financial, and spiritual issues may demand attention, and they often must be resolved under severe time constraints. Conflicts rise to the surface, and squabbles may break out between otherwise close and compatible family members. This is a poor time to be making important decisions, but it's precisely the moment when such decisions must be made. This is why it's better to have dealt in advance with as many difficult issues as possible.

Another stress factor is the current U.S. health care system. Most of us feel buffeted and sometimes manipulated by its complex bureaucracy—with the rules, regulations, and directives coming from multiple sources, almost of all of which are new to us. The intricacies (some would say the irrationality) of our system make it difficult to navigate. At a state legislative hearing, I once asked a roomful of health care "experts" to raise their hand if they could accurately predict how much a hospital visit for a routine illness might cost and how much they'd have to pay out of pocket to the hospital, doctors, and pharmacy after insurance covered its share. Not one hand went up.

This uncertainty is especially true when it comes to serious illness or injury. We trust and hope that the health care system will manage things and make us better, and it often does, even if later, when the paperwork hits, we are at a loss to understand all of what's going on.

Advance directives offer something rare and important in our modern medical system: they provide an opportunity to exert influence. This empowerment in itself is often comforting. It's like being at sea in a small boat: you can't control the weather and waves, but it's good to have a rudder with which to guide your course.

I once thought of subtitling this book "Take Control of the End of Your Life . . . Please," playing off the classic Henny Youngman joke. But it's true. When you take control of the end of your life, everyone is better off. As a doctor, I don't want to be put in the position of making tough decisions without the benefit of knowing what my patients want. And as a legislator, I'd prefer to work to empower people rather than have government micromanage private medical affairs.

It may seem difficult at first to tackle this project: getting the advance directive forms, thinking about them, talking about them with others, completing them, and storing them appropriately. But if you do, you will find yourself breathing a deep sigh of relief when it's over. You'll know that you've done the right thing, specifying choices according to your own personal beliefs; that you've spared others anguish and struggle; and that you've made decisions about the medical care you'll receive, decisions that will be honored. You'll be happy you did it.

In this book I discuss these issues by sharing stories from my medical practice and by offering my experience as a state legislator and a faculty member at the Johns Hopkins Bloomberg School of

Public Health. My goal is to put you in charge of your care in a way that matches your sensibilities and wishes. The end of life is more than a final diagnosis, more than a "cause of death" on a government certificate, more than legal forms or paperwork. Nowadays, it has become an exploration of circumstances and decisions that previously few people have ever had the chance to consider.

While it's true that no one gets out of here alive, our ability to contemplate the dying process has profound implications. Like all journeys, it begins with that first step and attention to little details. But the issue opens us to the breadth and scope of the human enterprise. Join me as we start out.

# 1

# The Basics

## Life, Death, Planning

A belief in hell and the knowledge that every ambition is doomed to frustration at the hands of a skeleton have never prevented the majority of human beings from behaving as though death were no more than an unfounded rumor.

ALDOUS HUXLEY

## Death Can Be Postponed but Not Canceled

Death is a subject that most people find difficult to talk about, particularly their own. As a member of the Maryland legislature, I've found people more willing to discuss tax hikes, gang wars, or raw sewage releases than this universal biological fact. Even bringing up the subject often brands the speaker as morbid. Yet despite the superb medical care available in the United States, our death rate remains the same as that of the poorest nation on earth: one per person.

Our fascination with violence in books, television, and movies is well documented. Some have suggested that we like to experience death at a safe distance—in a murder mystery or slasher flick. We're open to it as long as we can control it—by closing the book or turning off the picture. Our euphemisms for death are numerous: the grim reaper, deep six, big sleep, great beyond, buying the farm, kicking the bucket, pushing up daisies. Talking about it in euphemisms and slang makes it easier.

But when death gets personal, it isn't so easy. It's certainly true that we're delaying death by living longer. When I started in medicine, it was unusual to see patients in their 90s. Yet during a recent emergency room (ER) shift, I counted four patients above the age of 85, six older than 90, and two over 100 years of age. It used to be that the ER staff would buzz when a patient over 100 would appear. Now, it's routine.

Life can be sustained—and quality life, too. It is said that "60 is the new 40," and people often get to have two or three careers. Folks don't wind down at age 65; many are just getting started on something new. But death is still waiting for us all.

By the time we reach middle age, most of us have experienced the pain caused by the death of a friend or family member. Yet most of us have never witnessed someone dying, or even seen a dead body that hadn't been embalmed and cosmetically presented. In this respect we differ dramatically from prior generations. I often think our modern estrangement from the reality of death and dying accounts for some of our culture's insatiable hunger for details about other people's deaths, particularly if they are violent: beheadings on videotape, mutilating car accidents, serial killers' crimes.

There can be benefits to opening our eyes to death. Many religious sages over the centuries have taught that contemplating their own death unlocked the path to spiritual awakening. Since ancient times, the end of life has inspired sublime poetry and art. And, in areas such as estate planning and life insurance policies, there are financial benefits for our families when we look ahead to our own deaths.

But in our own unique era, when death can be delayed for decades through medical science, there is a further crucial benefit. By looking at the realities of death and dying we can make choices that will allow us and our loved ones to find that "best of both worlds," where life is prolonged and its inevitable end is as comfortable, conscious, and supported as possible.

Today we are living longer and better. This is because of major progress in public health and sanitation as well as significant medical advances in diagnostic tests (MRIs, CT and PET scans, etc.), treatments, devices, pharmaceuticals, and biotechnology. Sometimes we forget how far we've come in such a short time.

For example, when I was a medical resident, getting a CT scan almost required an act of Congress. Not many machines were available, maybe only a few for an entire city. Plus, the scans that came back were primitive. Nonetheless, we physicians were fascinated with the new cutting-edge technology. Today, meticulously detailed CT scans are routine and done everywhere, including in doctors' offices.

Consider the advances in the care of newborns. In 1963 President John F. Kennedy and his wife, Jacqueline, had a son, Patrick. He was born prematurely, weighing only 4 lbs. 10 oz. Despite the best medical care available, he died two days later of respiratory distress syndrome. Today, neonates who weigh less than half that amount regularly survive and thrive.

It used to be fairly rare for someone to survive a heart attack. Twenty to 30 years ago treatment consisted primarily of oxygen and bed rest. Now we have clot-busting drugs, medicines to stop fatal arrhythmias, implantable pacemakers, and cardiac surgery. Heart attacks, once a harbinger of imminent death, are now treated aggressively, and many patients live on for decades.

Certain cancers, once fatal, now are routinely treated. For example, many people survive lymphoma. Children with childhood leukemias, both acute lymphocytic leukemia and acute myelogenous leukemia, now have survival rates from 50 to 80 percent. A few years ago, youngsters with those diseases died quickly and painfully.

But all this progress also created a state of limbo. Our bodies can be made to live a bit longer, but when does brain death occur? It's easier to support the plumbing (heart, kidneys, blood vessels) than to keep the brain functioning at peak level.

And even in brain function, progress is being made. Recent advances in hypothermia (lowering body temperature) suggest that there are ways to protect the brain when circulation fails. A brain deprived of blood or oxygen for 3 to 5 minutes undergoes irreparable damage. But with a lower body temperature, the brain enters a state of hibernation and can recover when the temperature is later raised to normal levels. Much more research is needed to define the best ways to induce hypothermia, but again, it's safe to predict that new therapies will emerge.

Of course, in the end we will all die of something. And it is not always death that we fear, but rather the unknown process of dying. How will I meet my end? What will happen to me? Will I be in pain? Will death come swiftly and surely? Or will it drag out, slowly and miserably? We can't know in advance.

In our exploration of what the dying process may possibly entail and how advanced planning can help in difficult situations, I'm going share some stories. Some are well-known public cases. In others the names and other identifiers have been changed, but they are based on my real-life experience as a physician. These stories are not always comfortable to read, but they are accurate descriptions of what happens in today's medical world. Each illustrates a different aspect of end-of-life care and the decisions surrounding it, and each is followed by a discussion of the relevant aspects of the advance directive process.

## How Can We Know the Right Choice?

In January 2006, Ariel Sharon, the prime minister of Israel, suffered a massive stroke. He was rushed to the hospital, where he underwent three brain surgeries over the following days. His life was saved, but despite the best care available in the world, he never regained consciousness. During the following months he had major bowel and heart operations, as well as treatments for a kidney infection and pneumonia. The therapies succeeded, but, even years later, Mr. Sharon still had not regained consciousness.

Is there a chance that Mr. Sharon will ever return to a semblance of normal life? Is he truly getting "care," or has he become simply a collection of organs that are kept going by artificial means? Will he continue, with round-the-clock nursing care, to manage each of his bodily functions until some final and fatal event occurs? It's impossible to predict with 100 percent certainty, but it is extremely unlikely that Ariel Sharon will ever regain consciousness, much less a normal life.

Sharon's case is a dramatic and well-known one. But similar dramas are taking place every day throughout the United States. Modern medicine has put some people into a health care limbo where, like Ariel Sharon, they hover between life and death. This state can last for years.

The line between life and death is a fine one. Even the best doctors cannot predict with certainty the outcome in any given medical case. Individuals respond differently to treatment. Infections and cancerous growths are often unpredictable. New therapies are continually being discovered, so a condition that's currently untreatable may become treatable next year.

When patients are comatose, it's impossible to know what they would want. How can we find out what hurts and what is helpful? Is there a way to learn how they would like to be taken care of? How can we best prepare for unpredictable situations?

If it were you, what would you want in your last hours, days, weeks, or months of life? What sort of care? What fits your personal worldview, life perspective, religion, and spiritual values?

These questions are not easy to answer, but they are well worth pondering. In order to address them, we must begin with a consideration of our own ideas and experiences of death.

## Two Personal Experiences

I remember the first time I saw a dead person. It was in 1970 at Highland General Hospital in Oakland, California.

A friend of mine was on the straight-and-narrow path to go to medical school and become a doctor, something he'd always planned to do. In order to increase his chances of acceptance to med school, he decided to volunteer at a local hospital emergency room.

I, on the other hand, was ending my college career at the University of California, Berkeley, without clear direction. I was a history major, but I was open to new experiences, so when Robert mentioned his plan and invited me to join him, I accepted.

Our duties consisted of bringing coffee to patients and staff, carrying blood tubes to the lab, and generally doing little tasks to help the place run better. For me, it was the first time I ever had the chance to chat with a physician without being a patient. One doctor took a few minutes to explain the concept of an electrocardiogram (EKG), and I was fascinated and inspired. This looked like the combination of science skills and humanitarian values that was right for me.

One evening an ambulance screeched to a halt at the ER entry, and the crew wheeled in a middle-aged African American woman undergoing cardio-pulmonary resuscitation (CPR). The ER became a flurry of activity. I stood in the back and peered between the nurses, doctors, and other staff as they tried to revive the patient. After about 30 minutes, it was clear that the resuscitation had failed. The lead doctor halted the proceedings and noted the time of death.

Just as quickly as it had filled with people and machines, now the room emptied. During the few minutes before a nurse's aide came to clean the body and transport it to the hospital morgue, I found myself alone with the deceased. I stood in the corner for a minute, and then slowly approached the gurney that held the body. I looked at the woman and tried to discern the difference between life and death. After some hesitation, I reached out and gently touched her. No response. Again, and no response. I don't know why I did this. For some reason, her obvious condition was not obvious to me. She looked fine, and yet she was dead. Before I left the room I mentally thanked her for allowing me to be present at her passing.

That experience has stayed with me to this day.

Max Mont was my stepfather and a truly remarkable individual. He married my mother when I was 9. Max devoted his life to social change. He read widely and was fully informed on world history, politics, and culture. As director of the Jewish Labor Committee in Los Angeles, he worked for the rights of exploited garment workers and farm workers, for unions, for fair housing, and for fair employment laws in California. He built coalitions between disparate groups, and he was an integral part of many steps toward social progress from the 1950s to the 1980s.

As an adolescent, Max had been stricken with rheumatic fever that damaged his heart valves. Over the years the damage increased, and Max underwent several major cardiac operations, including a mitral valve replacement. He took excellent care of himself, watching his diet and weight and never smoking or drinking.

But finally the effect of the surgeries, medications, and recurrent illnesses took their toll. A massive hemorrhage required one kidney to be removed. Eventually the other kidney failed, and Max went on dialysis.

Dialysis limited Max, as it does all kidney patients. Going to a center three times a week for several hours at a time was exhausting and boring.

Max noticed that his mind was starting to fail as well as his body. His memory and alertness faded. He was sleeping more and found that concentrating on a task had become impossible. He could no longer stay focused enough to read or write. For a man who had lived such an active life of the mind, this was devastating.

By that time, I had left California and moved to Maryland. I had been a doctor for over 15 years. My wife Shelley and I started our family, and I was busy at work as chairman of the Emergency Medicine Department at a large suburban hospital.

One day, Max called to tell me that he had made the decision not to return to dialysis. He knew that stopping dialysis would mean the end, and he wanted me to come to Los Angeles to be with him.

When I arrived, my mother and Max and I had a long talk. He looked gaunt and worn out. He explained that for him life was no longer worth living. He couldn't do anything except stay in bed, sleeping through most of each day. It would take all his strength to rouse himself from his stupor for a few minutes, and then he'd collapse again. Dialysis had worn him out, and he could see that the course of his life would be relentlessly downhill. He knew there was no recovery possible, just more of the same, gradually becoming worse. He wanted to make some decisions while he was still capable of doing so.

The next week was intense. Max's closest friends came to his bedside to pay their respects. Sometimes they just sat by, and sometimes they discussed old times. There were tears and laughter. My mother and I managed the flow of people. By the fifth day the flow of visitors diminished to a trickle, and toward the end just the two of us took care of Max.

As the toxins in his blood built up, his waking moments decreased dramatically. Max was more somnolent than alert. He stopped eating, occasionally requesting sips of water but no more.

We had some codeine pain pills and Valium, and we gave these to Max when he was in pain or became agitated. He began to slide in and out of awareness, but he was always comfortable and comforted. We stayed with him continuously, and his last days and hours were peaceful.

At the end, his breathing became slower and shallower, then slower and shallower still. We weren't quite sure when he would take his last breath, but finally it was clear that he was dead.

Max had made arrangements to have his body donated to the University of California, Los Angeles, Medical School. There were things to be learned from his diseased heart and the condition of his artificial valve, and the hope that a researcher would discover something that would help other patients in the future.

When my mother and I finished saying our final goodbyes, we called UCLA, and a team arrived to take Max away.

Max gave me much, not only in life, but in death. I reflected on his process of dying, so different from the intense activity I knew as a physician. In the hospital, we struggled to keep people going, often long past the time that we knew would offer any hope of meaningful recovery. People died tied to machines and monitors, in the company of strangers, with loved ones kept in the waiting room.

I often was the one who had to go out and break the bad news. Sometimes there were intensely emotional reactions. I understood this when a death was unexpected or sudden, but it struck me as odd that people would become hysterical when the deceased had been suffering from advanced cancer or clearly terminal heart failure.

This was in stark contrast to what I experienced with Max. His death was calm, reassuring, and natural. He had time to make his farewells, and he died at home with family. For those of us left behind, it gave us a chance to say goodbye, to let go of him gradually. It somehow helped to make the pain of his loss more bearable.

Sometimes, as with the woman who died in that Oakland ER, there are no choices available. People tried their best to save her life, and her loved ones had to deal with the suddenness of their loss as best they could. But when a disease or injury allows us a choice, as in Max's case, it is helpful to have considered these issues in advance of the crisis.

# 2

# Controversies and How to Avoid Becoming One

Die? I should say not, dear fellow. No Barrymore would allow
such a conventional thing to happen to him.

JOHN BARRYMORE

## Red Herrings and Legitimate Issues

Often discussions of end-of-life issues revolve around certain highly
charged scenarios, covered extensively by the media. My personal
belief is that these controversies, while fascinating, are often distrac-
tions from more serious and universal issues. Yet at other times they
can raise important questions for all of us.

### Assisted Suicide

This is when one person helps another to actively end his or her life.
It can include anything from providing a potentially lethal dose of
medicine all the way to fully participating in a suicide. Dr. Jack
Kevorkian brought this issue to public attention in a sensational-
ized way. Three states (Oregon, Washington, and Montana) allow
physician-assisted suicide under certain very narrow circumstances.

*Nothing in this book relates to assisted suicide.* There are appropriate and legal ways in which individuals can direct their care
without having to resort to problematic measures that raise complex ethical and legal issues. An important point: assisted suicide
does *not* include the case of a person who chooses to forego treatment and die a natural death when there is no expectation of
recovery.

### "Death Panels"

This issue arose in the summer of 2009 as the debate on health care reform got underway. Some opponents of reform mistakenly argued that a section of the proposed law would create "death panels" and that government would be "pulling the plug on Granny." Having read that section of the bill, I saw nothing to justify such extreme claims. Basically, the proposal would allow physicians to be reimbursed by Medicare for taking the time to discuss end-of-life care with patients who requested it. This is one of the most important conversations a patient and physician can have, and it should be paid for, just as you pay for other time spent with your doctor.

### Pain Medicine: Narcotics, Tranquilizers, and Medical Marijuana

There are a variety of medicines used to treat people with serious and advanced illnesses. Sometimes they are given to help patients endure difficult treatments or side effects. Sometimes they are used to relieve the discomfort that may come as part of the dying process. Patients and their families may be anxious about using these medicines, fearful of addiction, dependency, side effects, and oversedation. These concerns are legitimate, but all can be addressed.

#### Narcotics

Narcotics, also known as opiates, are a class of drugs that relieve pain very effectively. Some common ones are codeine, morphine, fentanyl, hydromorphone (Dilaudid), and oxycodone (OxyContin). Versions of this class of drugs have also been abused, especially heroin, which provides a dangerously tempting "rush" as well as pain relief. However, when pharmaceutically approved drugs are used *carefully* for pain management, their addictive potential may be kept under control. In fact, once pain is managed, the doses can often be reduced. There are side effects, as happens with almost any medicine, and the most common ones with opiates are constipation and sleepiness. But again, with careful dosing these can be minimized.

Opiates can be given by mouth, by skin patch, or by injection. Each person may have a preferred method of administration. These medicines can be safely taken at home, or in a hospital, nursing home, or hospice. But, however given, these drugs pretty much work the same way.

I had one patient who was in mild to moderate pain almost constantly, and he resisted the use of narcotics. He was depressed and had trouble performing at work. However, he finally gave in and was started on morphine. Almost immediately, his pain was relieved and he began to sleep better. His mood lightened and his thinking improved. He functioned better in every aspect of life, and he later told me that he wished he'd started a pain-relief program sooner.

Sometimes our emotions around accepting death get entangled in the decision to use narcotics for pain relief. After all, what are the risks when a patient is at the end of life? Is there a need to worry about addiction when someone has only a few months to live?

### Tranquilizers

Sedatives and tranquilizers are another set of medications that may be prescribed. They can help with anxiety, sleep, and mood disorders—all common symptoms in those with serious illness—and, when used responsibly, the benefits outweigh the risks.

Of course, there are important nonpharmacologic methods of managing pain and anxiety, including acupuncture, prayer, meditation, massage, music and art therapy, and others. As treatments options, these should be considered equally with standard medications. In fact, I believe that all modalities should be used. They are often complementary and work together well in ways we may not appreciate. All patients should have the opportunity to find what works best for them individually.

In optimal situations, patients with an advanced illness are getting the benefit of being taken care of by a team of professionals, including doctors, nurses, and pharmacists. When that is the case, just about every pain and anxiety condition can be safely managed.

## Medical Marijuana

The issue of medical marijuana—a third category of pain medications for serious illnesses and end-of-life scenarios—is in the headlines. Seventeen states have made medical marijuana available in some manner, and a number of others are considering doing the same. On the federal level marijuana is still illegal, which has made research difficult, though not impossible.

Some background may help here. Many medications come from plants. Besides the opiates mentioned above, there are many others that originate in the plant world, such as digitalis, penicillin, aspirin, and quinine. Seen in that context, marijuana should be treated like any other medication. It has its uses and side effects, with reasons to start the drug and reasons to stop.

Unfortunately, our country has a history of irrational marijuana phobia that, for some, remains out of proportion to the drug's risks. I've read numerous studies and am convinced that there is a place for marijuana to be used to help patients who can't be helped otherwise. Yes, there are dangers, as there are with just about every other medicine.

With any powerful medication, it's not the drug that matters so much as the context of its use. Let's say a person is in possession of 30 OxyContin pills. If the drug was obtained illegally or by subterfuge, with the intention of selling it to addicts, then the use of the drug in that context is inappropriate. But if the person has widespread cancer with severe bone pain, then possession of the medication is entirely appropriate.

The federal government, through the Drug Enforcement Agency (DEA), classifies certain medications having a risk of abuse into categories. These are called Schedules 1 to 5, with 1 being the most dangerous. Schedule 1 includes medications that are considered to have very high risks and no proven benefits. Drugs in this class include heroin, LSD, and marijuana. Schedule 2 drugs are those with significant risks but also significant uses. This category of drugs consists of the stronger narcotics, amphetamines, and cocaine (used to stop bleeding and reduce pain for some surgeries). Schedule 3 drugs comprise milder narcotics, like hydrocodone/acetaminophen (Lortab) and paracetamol/acetaminophen (Tylenol #3), as well as anabolic (body-building) steroids that have other, legitimate medical uses. Also on that list is dronabinol (Marinol), an oral form of THC, which is thought to be the main active ingredient in marijuana. To round out the DEA's list, Schedule 4 includes the most common tranquilizers and sleeping pills, like diazepam (Valium); Schedule 5 contains very mild narcotics, such as those found in cough syrup.

Does marijuana belong in the same category as heroin and LSD? Most would agree that while marijuana is not a risk-free drug, its risks are nowhere near as dangerous as the drugs with which it has been classed. I believe the DEA should move marijuana from Schedule 1 to Schedule 2. Classified appropriately, pharmaceutical companies would then enter the market and create a standardized product that doctors could prescribe and pharmacists could fill. But until the federal government acts, state legislatures have moved to safeguard their citizens' rights to obtain medication that can help treat certain serious conditions. This process will continue, as polls show that over 80 percent of Americans favor controlled medical marijuana use.

One of those Americans recently testified before the Maryland state legislature at a bill hearing in Annapolis. Debbie M. is a 55-year-old chemist, the mother of three, who developed chronic myelogenous leukemia. Four years ago, she underwent a bone marrow transplant at Johns Hopkins Hospital. After 60 days in isolation, struggling to take 17 medications per day, she grew progressively weaker and sicker. Such a downhill course is a known possibility with bone marrow transplants. Medical professionals sometime refer to it as "circling the drain." The fear is that while the cancer will be cured, the patient will die from the treatment and its side effects.

Everything had been tried to curb Debbie's nausea and increase her appetite, but she simply could not eat and was wasting away to skin and bones. Finally, the possibility of using marijuana was raised.

Her Hopkins oncologist could only shrug. "I can't officially recommend it, but you can do whatever you feel you must."

Somehow marijuana was obtained, meaning that somebody went out to the illegal drug market, took risks by committing a criminal act, and paid money to get a green, leafy substance advertised as marijuana. Without government controls, there is no way to know for sure if an illegal substance is genuine and unadulterated. Fortunately, in this case it was.

For two months Debbie smoked marijuana several times a week. As it helped to stimulate her appetite, she gained weight and slowly recovered. Today, she's doing fine. She never used marijuana before or since. She credits it with saving her life.

As another example, I took care of a patient in the ER who was on chemotherapy and arrived dehydrated, with intractable nausea. She wanted to tell me what she felt. "Doc," she said, "this is what it's like. Have you ever been really nauseated? You wouldn't know about pregnancy and morning sickness, but maybe in college you drank too much one night and woke up hung over with a horrible bellyache. Or maybe you got seasick or carsick. Or maybe you ate some bad food, and spent 24 hours not knowing whether to sit on the toilet to crap or look at it face down to puke. Remember how you felt? You couldn't do anything but feel sick. That's what I feel like, with nausea coming on in waves every few hours every day." Her vivid description made quite an impression on me, and she sensitized me to what some of my patients were going through.

Marijuana is not a cure-all, but it should be available for use, just as other medications are. Used judiciously, responsibly, carefully, and accountably, it can bring relief when nothing else works. Isn't that one of the most important goals in medicine?

We've been waging a war on drugs since 1970, and we can argue about whether or not it has been a success. But one thing we should all agree on: it's time to take the sick and dying off the battlefield. People in pain should not be held hostage to what I believe is an irrational political agenda.

## The Economics of End-of-Life Care

It may not seem polite to discuss financial considerations in end-of-life care, but this is another uncomfortable topic that can't be avoided. For most Americans today, it is estimated that 25 percent or more of all the health care dollars spent throughout their lives are doled out in the very last months of life. Money is expended keeping people alive far past any hope of reasonable recovery, money that could be spent earlier, when the impact would be much greater in terms of the quality and length of their lives.

Some worry that the use of advance directives for end-of-life planning is designed primarily to save money. Such planning probably will reduce health care costs for many people, although in some cases that won't be true. Personally, I believe that a person's wishes must always come first, and that economic impacts should be secondary.

The number and proportion of those over 65 in the United States is rising steadily. And with the baby boom generation about to hit old age, with its accompanying chronic diseases, it is inevitable that health care costs will increase.

According to the Congressional Research Service (CRS), more of us are dying in care facilities—in the hospital (58%) or nursing homes (20%)—than at home (22%). Expenses in institutions always cost more than at home. One question for us to address is what portion of the deaths in outside settings could be more reasonably managed at home? In fact, the CRS reports that family members of loved ones "who died at a private home with hospice services were more likely to report a favorable dying experience." Of patients in a hospice program, over 70 percent chose to die at home.

Who pays for this care? What about insurance coverage? Costs for end-of-life care may be paid by private insurance, Medicare, or Medicaid, or they can be self-paid. In fact, about one-fourth of all Medicare spending is for the last year of life, and over 50 percent of that is in an acute-care hospital. There are geographic variations as well. For example, Medicare spending for the end of life in New York, New Jersey, and California averages 20 percent above the national norm, while in North Dakota, South Dakota, and Iowa, it is 25 percent below. In the final analysis, we, as taxpayers, employers, and individuals, are all paying for this. Let's make sure we're paying for what we really want.

This is why completing an advance directive is so important, and why it plays such a key role. The very act of designating when, where, how, and how much care a person wants ends up defining not only the amount that will be spent, but the way in which those resources will be used.

## The Terri Schiavo Case

This case made headlines in 2004 and 2005. The State of Florida, and then the U.S. Congress, became involved in the care decisions of this unfortunate woman and in the conflicts within her family. Her situation (described in chapter 7) highlighted the issue of advance directives and living wills. Many people recognized that the entire controversy could have been avoided if Ms. Schiavo had completed an advance directive. In the wake of extensive news coverage, there was a surge in requests for the forms for these documents. Since then, however, the push for advance directives has quieted down.

## The Solution: Advance Directives—Making Our Wishes Known

The irony is that many aspects of the Schiavo controversy (and others) have already been addressed. The problem is that most Americans are either unaware of or have not taken advantage of the available tools.

In 1991, the Self-Determination Act was passed by the U.S. Congress and signed into law by the president. The act specifies that individuals have the right to medical decision making, including the right to accept or refuse treatment. The act permits individuals to create an advance directive to spell out these choices, and it requires health care facilities to provide information about advance directives when patients enter the system. Additionally, a facility cannot use the presence or absence of an advance directive to refuse care to a patient.

An advance directive is a straightforward way to designate end-of-life care decisions and make them work for you. Advance directives are legal documents, and they are available at no (or very little) cost. Some are online, like "Five Wishes," one of the most popular and readily accessible forms (www.agingwithdignity.org). Advance directives can be obtained from your attorney, your hospital, or your state government. At the end of this book you will find a state-by-state listing of resources where you can get this information.

The advance directive forms are easy to fill out. They are clear, well organized, and only a few pages long. Their main cost is in time: taking the time to think about what sort of care you want, should you ever be in a situation where you can't make medical decisions for yourself. You might want to talk about these choices with family and other advisors (doctors, clergy, lawyers), though this is not required. Fill out the form, file it in a safe place, give a copy to your health care provider, and let a few trusted people know where it is. That's it.

Advance directives typically consist of four parts:

1. *Choosing the kind of care you want*: This section has various names: a "Living Will," "Treatment Preferences," or "Instructions for Health Care." It will contain specific details about your medical treatment preferences and values.
2. *Choosing someone to act on your behalf when you cannot*: This is called a "Medical Power of Attorney," with the person you select referred to as a "Health Care Agent." If you become unable to make your own health care choices, this person will have the authority to do so for you.
3. *After-death instructions*: These include instructions about

organ or body donation, disposition of the body, and funeral arrangements.

4. *Documentation*: This refers to the process of having signatures and witnesses that will make sure your advance directive is legal and will be followed.

In the following chapters we'll discuss each of these elements in more detail. We'll also be looking at the specifics of death and dying. One day I hope that completing an advance directive will become as accepted and normal a responsibility as maintaining a driver's license, paying your taxes, or saving money for your retirement. Reading and thinking about such concrete details can sometimes be difficult, but you will need this information in order to make an informed judgment about your personal choices. Let's begin.

# 3

# Alberta Cole

## *Not Deciding Is a Decision*

It hath often been said, that it is not death, but dying, which is terrible.

HENRY FIELDING

When I met her, Alberta Cole was 92 years old and living in a nursing home. Born in West Virginia, she and her husband moved to Maryland after the Second World War, when he took a job in the steel mills. She raised three children and was the proud grandmother of six. A homemaker until her last child moved out, she went back to school to become a bookkeeper. When her husband fell seriously ill with emphysema in the 1990s, Alberta began working from home to care for him. In 2000 he died.

Alberta continued to live in her modest, three-bedroom family home in a working-class neighborhood, but she was becoming increasingly infirm herself. In 2001 Alberta fell while in the bathroom. Unable to get up, she lay on the floor for two days until her daughter Mary came to check on her and called 911. Alberta arrived in the emergency room bruised, dehydrated, and with a hip fracture. A CT scan of her head showed a small stroke.

Alberta's stay in the hospital was difficult. She became agitated in the evenings, something the staff recognized as "sundowning." This term refers to elderly patients who, when away from their familiar home environment, become disoriented and confused. Eventually, Alberta was discharged to a rehabilitation program in the hospital.

Her children visited Alberta through her hospital course. Daughter Mary, herself in her late 60s, lived nearby and came most often. Her son Paul and other daughter Clare lived out of town and visited when they could.

Although the hospital staff ascertained that Alberta had no advance directive and offered her the form, she was too distraught by her pain and disorientation to complete it. Her children doubted it was necessary. After all, hadn't the doctors and nurses done all they could for Alberta? Wouldn't that continue to be the case?

Eventually Alberta was able to go home, and a visiting nurse was arranged for Mondays, Wednesdays, and Fridays. Alberta's mobility was impaired, and she struggled to move around the house or complete basic chores such as shopping. She became increasingly disheveled and withdrawn. On one visit the nurse observed that Alberta looked weak and pale and had a fever. She called for a private ambulance that took Alberta to the emergency room.

In the ER it was noted that Alberta had multiple problems, the main one being a urinary tract infection. In addition, she had early symptoms of a skin breakdown on her low back, a consequence of too much sitting. And perhaps worst of all, Alberta showed definite signs of increasing dementia. She was now 90 years old. She knew her name and the city she lived in, but she could not give her street address. She knew she was in a hospital but didn't know its name, even though she had been there many times before, including when taking care of her husband. She didn't know the date, the day of the week, or the year.

This hospitalization lasted four days. Alberta received intravenous antibiotics, physical therapy, and a complete mental health evaluation. It was very difficult to assess the state of her competency to make decisions. Finally, she was stable enough for discharge. But to where could she safely be discharged?

Although Alberta was insistent on returning home, her daughter Mary felt that was too risky. Lacking the resources to care for Alberta in her own home, Mary tried to persuade her mother to go to an assisted living center, assuming an affordable one could be found. The other siblings were not available for discussion. Ultimately Alberta's persistence won out, and she was discharged home with careful instructions, an aide for in-home care, and a visiting nurse.

But this lasted only a few weeks. Alberta did not fare well. Both her home aide and visiting nurse tried to persuade her to make a doctor's visit, but Alberta was increasingly hostile and resistant. She had angry outbursts, and once she even took a swing at the nurse.

Another visit to the ER ensued when the home aide found Alberta collapsed in her bedroom. The ER note started "LOL FOF"—which means "Little old lady, found on floor." That abbreviation is a stark indication of the frequency of emergency room patients in similar circumstances.

This led to a 10-day hospitalization. A CT scan showed multi-infarct dementia, meaning many small strokes had taken their toll on her brain. Alberta's heart, lungs, and digestive system were functioning normally, but she again had a urinary tract infection. Intravenous fluids and antibiotics were given, in addition to antianxiety medications to manage her frequent screams and outbursts. Sometimes restraints were used at night to keep Alberta from falling out of bed. This is a particularly unpleasant procedure, for patients and staff.

Both social work and psychiatric consultations were requested, but before those could happen, Alberta suffered a cardiac arrest while being taken for an x-ray.

Alberta's medical code status (regarding resuscitation) had never been determined. She was not wearing a bracelet indicating "no CPR," that being shorthand for cardio-pulmonary resuscitation. Her chart was not marked in any way that has become standard when end-of-life decisions have been made. Because she was not designated as "no CPR," by default she was automatically made a "full code" patient.

Since staff was with her immediately, CPR was started. This involved a hard thump to the chest, followed by cardiac compressions. Most people know what cardiac compressions are, at least from having seen this on TV. But to do it is hard work. Both hands are placed on the sternum (breastbone), and by rocking up and down, the sternum is depressed. This helps compress the heart and keep the blood circulating. It also leads to broken ribs at the point where the ribs join the breastbone. Sometimes, when doing CPR, you can feel the ribs snap and crack and then crunch on each succeeding chest compression.

An oxygen mask was placed on Alberta's face while preparations were made for intubation. This involves putting a plastic tube about 18 inches long and 3/4 of an inch wide into the patient's windpipe. First, any dentures or false teeth are removed. Then a laryngoscope is used, a metal tool about 6 inches long and 3 inches wide that pulls open the mouth, sweeps the tongue aside, and opens up the whole oral cavity so the operator (usually a physician, or sometimes a respiratory therapist) can see the patient's vocal cords. Sometimes patients vomit during the procedure, so suction equipment is used to remove the chunks and liquid. Medications are given by vein to paralyze the patient if that person is awake or has a tightly clenched jaw, or if the patient's anatomy makes the procedure difficult. Sometimes intubation happens quickly and easily. At other times, it's a trying and difficult process. Once the vocal cords are seen, the tube is swiftly jammed between them into the windpipe, and the outside end is connected to a respirator.

The tube in Alberta's windpipe made it impossible for her to speak. On top of baseline dementia, the medications used to ease her pain and anxiety, as well as side effects of other drugs, clouded her mind even further. There was no way to communicate with Alberta or find out what she was thinking or feeling.

She was then transferred to the hospital's intensive care unit. She spent three days there and made a slow recovery. Here are some of the basic procedures that were done, which are standard practice in ICUs.

A catheter (plastic tube) was placed into her bladder, both to monitor urine output and to prevent self-soiling. This involves a lubricated tube about the size of a soda straw being threaded up through the urinary tract into the bladder. For the practitioner, this is a relatively easy procedure, especially in a female patient. In male patients, it can be more difficult, because the catheter must often pass through an enlarged prostate gland. For both male and female patients, this is likely to be an invasive and uncomfortable experience.

Nutrition was given to Alberta via a plastic tube that was inserted through her nose and into her stomach. I've placed plenty of these, and, while it is not a particularly difficult technique, patients generally hate it. We use nasal spray first to shrink the tissues inside the nose, and anesthetic lubricants can ease the passage of the tube, but no matter how it's done, it's a tough procedure to endure. Infrequently the naso-gastric (NG) tube goes into the windpipe or coils up in the patient's esophagus. Because of this, after every insertion steps are taken to ensure that the tube is correctly positioned. If incorrectly placed, the procedure must be repeated until done successfully.

Intravenous medications and fluids of all types were given to Alberta and carefully balanced to help her recovery and avoid complications. To give intravenous fluids, IVs (intravenous tubes of thin plastic) are established by putting a needle into the patient's vein, sliding the tube over the needle, taping it down, and then removing the needle. Many of us have been on the receiving end of IVs when giving blood or getting fluids or medicine by vein, so we know what it's like to be jabbed by a needle. Like all procedures, sometimes this goes quickly and easily, and sometimes not. When dealing with very elderly patients who have been in the hospital before, it often becomes increasingly difficult to find a usable vein. Nurses are very adept at locating veins, and while the arms and hands are the first choice, sometimes IVs are placed in the feet or legs, or the superficial veins of the neck. When no sites are found, then more invasive procedures are needed. More on that later.

On day four in the ICU, the tube in Alberta's windpipe was removed, and she went to the step-down unit.

Alberta was debilitated: her heart, kidneys, and liver had been damaged. These organs were functioning, but in a limited way. Her level of awareness was impossible to gauge, but it was becoming obvious that the right side of her body was weaker than the left. The neurologist's note pointed out that this meant that the left side of her brain (which controls the right side of the body) had been damaged by a stroke. This also meant that Alberta's use of language was limited, as the location of that function is also in the left side of the brain. Hence communication, already difficult, became almost completely impossible.

Nutrition was needed. At first, this was done via the NG-tube, but a tube like that cannot be left in for more than a few days. Thus the decision was now made to place a G-tube in her body. The "G" stands for gastric, meaning stomach. Alberta was taken to the operating room. There the surgeon created a hole in her abdominal wall, directly into her stomach. The feeding tube was pushed in and held in place by a balloon in her stomach. Once secured, liquid nutrition can be poured directly into the stomach via a G-tube.

By day eight it was time to start to decide where to send Alberta next. Plus, the utilization review (UR) process was beginning. UR involves insurance companies and their in-hospital representatives (usually nurses) who review the care of patients. The goal is to shorten hospital stays and thus limit the company's financial exposure. If a patient stays in the hospital too long, the insurance company can refuse to pay for the extra days, meaning the hospital or the patient may have to absorb the extra costs. Sometimes, this amounts to thousands of dollars. The hospital counters this process with its own UR committee. This committee does battle with the insurance company if it disagrees with the company's payment denial. In the best of circumstances, the UR nurse and the hospital's UR committee cooperate with the patient's attending physician, the person most responsible for the patient's care. The attending physician, in turn, is pushed by several competing forces: what's best for the patient, the family's needs and resources, fear of liability for any wrong decision, and self-interest in getting paid.

The hospital's social work team got involved in Alberta's situation, as it invariably does in these sorts of cases. Alberta's family was contacted. Mary, the oldest, felt her mother just wanted to "die in peace." But Paul wasn't sure. Clare, who, up to this point, had left most decisions in Mary's hands, suddenly became concerned. She insisted that her mother "get the best of care—everything should be done to save her." Clare forcefully pushed for her point of view and implied that she would consider getting an attorney to make sure that what she wanted was done. So Alberta was not moved to a "No CPR" status.

In the meantime, several local nursing homes were contacted, and on her 10th day of hospitalization, a bed in one of them was found for Alberta. A private ambulance company transported her there from the hospital.

To pay for the nursing home, both Medicare (the federal program for seniors) and Medicaid (the federal program for the lowest income people) were contacted. Alberta's assets were too great for her to qualify for Medicaid. Thus the "spend down" process began. Alberta's assets, accumulated over a lifetime, were slowly dissipated so that she could eventually be poor enough to qualify for Medicaid. What might have been an inheritance evaporated quickly, as nursing home care costs thousands of dollars per month.

In the nursing home, Alberta received "as good care as was possible," meaning that it was inconsistent. The nursing home, also under continuous pressures, was always in a struggle to attract and retain quality staff. When staff members were good, they were very good, but when they were bad, they were horrid.

Alberta's days consisted of lying in bed. She had to be turned frequently to avoid bedsores. A word first about bedsores. This is a condition where the skin breaks down into red areas that can become actual open wounds. They can vary from the size of a dime to several inches across. Bedsores can become infected, draining pus, and these infections can take weeks to months to cure—when they are cured at all. When all else fails, skin grafts may be required to close the open wound, but even this doesn't always work.

Bedsores are something every nursing home and chronic-care facility struggles to avoid in their patients, but sometimes they are unavoidable. Even Christopher Reeve, the superstar actor who suffered total-body paralysis from the neck down and who had the very best care money could buy, eventually developed bedsores. These sores contributed to his death.

The nursing staff did all they could to keep Alberta from developing bedsores, but sores eventually appeared. Bandages and medications were placed on them, and although the sores did not get bigger, they didn't shrink, either.

On good days, Alberta was put in a wheelchair and placed in the hallway. She would sit and stare at the traffic of patients, their families, and staff. Often she'd fall asleep in the chair, slump over, and then be taken back to her room. Or she'd be taken to the TV room and lined up with other patients in front of the TV, which was tuned to daytime game shows or soap operas.

She wore a diaper and needed to be cleaned two to four times each day. Daughter Mary's visits were daily at first, until this became too demanding for her, as she had her own medical problems. Paul tried to come weekly, and he usually did on Saturdays, spending an hour with his mother. Clare came intermittently, sometimes not for a month or two, and then, if in town, daily for a few days. During these visits, she'd want to meet with the nursing director and Alberta's doctor to go over details of Alberta's care plan.

Over the following six months, Alberta became increasingly immobile. Her joints became stiff, especially in her right arm and leg. These limbs developed contractures, meaning that they slowly became frozen in a flexed position. Alberta was bedridden 24 hours a day.

A urinary catheter had now been in place for weeks. As so often happens, a urinary infection developed. This was first evident when Alberta spiked a low-grade fever and the staff noticed that the urine in her collection bag looked cloudy. Alberta's doctor prescribed antibiotics, and these were added to her medication regimen. But her condition did not improve, and one evening Alberta's blood pressure was found to be dropping.

Paramedics were called to the nursing home, and the ambulance arrived at 11 p.m. After several jabs, an intravenous line was placed, fluids were given, and Alberta was taken to the emergency room.

In the ER, the hospital's nursing staff drew blood and urine for numerous tests. After the doctor's examination, x-rays and an EKG were ordered, and fluids and antibiotics were given by vein. However, Alberta's veins were fragile and bruised, and the veins "blew," meaning that fluid was going into the soft tissues around the IV site and not into the bloodstream. Therefore, the ER doctor decided to insert a central line, a large IV placed directly into a large vein located deep below the skin. This would ensure that fluids and medicines were going to the right place.

The three most common areas for a central line are the groin (femoral vein), neck (jugular vein), and chest (subclavian vein). In Alberta's case, the doctor chose the subclavian route. The skin in her right upper chest was prepped with an antiseptic solution and then numbed with an injection of lidocaine. Using sterile technique and with careful attention to avoid puncturing vital organs, the doctor first probed her chest with a large needle (attached to a syringe) until the correct vein was punctured. During a central-line procedure, this is detected when blood quickly fills the syringe. Then the syringe is removed and a metal guide wire is inserted through the needle. Next, the needle is withdrawn over the guide wire, and the skin is nicked open with a scalpel at the point where the wire enters the skin. A stiff plastic tube (called a dilator) is passed over the guide wire to spread open the tissues and create a wider hole in the vein. The dilator is then removed, usually with a gush of blood, leaving a tubular track in its place. This allows the intravenous catheter to be advanced over the guide wire into the vein. The wire is removed, and the catheter is then stitched into place.

This procedure is commonly done in ERs, and I have performed it hundreds of times. Sometimes it goes quickly and easily, and the whole process takes less than 20 minutes. Sometimes it is difficult, and requires repeated searching for the vein. At other times there are complications, such as puncturing an artery or a lung during the procedure. On occasion, the patient develops an infection a day or two later.

With Alberta's central line in place, fluids and medicines were given, and blood was drawn for more testing. After 3 hours, all the test results were back. These confirmed the diagnosis of a urinary tract infection that had spread to the bloodstream. An hour later the ER physician and Alberta's regular doctor discussed the case and decided to admit Alberta to the hospital. Because the hospital was nearly full, Alberta stayed in the ER for 10 more hours until her bed was ready. She did not seem aware of anything going on around her, so she probably was unaware of the delay.

During the next three days, Alberta's condition gradually improved. Because her infection was caused by bacteria that had become resistant to routine antibiotics, more advanced ones were needed. Drug resistance is a real problem for many reasons, including overuse of antibiotics and recurrent infections in patients who are in and out of hospitals and nursing homes. On day four of this hospital stay, Alberta was without fever and back to her baseline function, meaning lying in bed, moaning occasionally, sleeping most of the time, and sometimes being restrained to prevent her from pulling out the various tubes.

Back when I was a resident physician-in-training in the 1970s, I often worked in the intensive care unit. I remember an elderly man, severely ill and chronically debilitated. He was dying of heart, lung, and kidney failure, with all their complications. He was on a respirator. He was very weak, but every day, mustering all his strength and will, he would slowly move his right hand from his side up to his neck, where the respirator tube was connected to his tracheotomy (a hole in the front of his neck into the trachea, where the tube was inserted). This would take hours, as his hand could only move inch by inch. When he'd reach the tube, he'd work to disconnect it—a suicide attempt. He wanted to end his suffering, and this was the only way in which he could communicate his wish. After the first few times, the staff realized what was happening. As soon as the agonizing effort once more brought his hand near the tube, a nurse or resident physician would run over, quickly pull his hand down to foil his effort, and the process would start all over again. This patient's attending physician was famous for never "giving up" on his patients. He subjected them to every conceivable treatment, long after any hope of recovery was possible. It was as if he considered stopping treatment—no matter how painful or invasive—to be a professional defeat. Of course, after a couple of weeks of this tragic performance, nature took its course, and the man died.

Because there was no advance medical directive in Alberta's case, she was kept alive through two more episodes like the one above. One involved another urinary tract infection, and the other resulted from her bedsores (now large and draining yellow, foul-smelling pus). Each consisted of a hospital admission, a central line, and intravenous drugs. There was one brief cardiac arrest, from which she was resuscitated with electric cardioversion. Finally, she developed pneumonia and again was sent to the hospital. After one day in the ICU, her heart stopped beating. Because her code status was not clear or specified, full CPR was given. Multiple electric shocks, medications, and chest compressions (with accompanying broken ribs) failed to revive her. After 40 minutes, the code was "called" (meaning ended), and Alberta was declared dead.

Twenty-two months had elapsed from her first hospitalization to her last. From an economic perspective, Alberta's hospital costs were over $60,000, and her nursing home care ran about $4000 per month. The total, well over $150,000, was much more than the entirety of Alberta's health care expenses during all the previous years of her life.

More importantly, what was the human cost? Is there a way to quantify Alberta's suffering? She underwent multiple invasive procedures and suffered from their complications. She endured numerous transfers between her home, the ER, the operating room, the ICU, a step-down unit, and her nursing home. Through it all she was unable to understand what was happening, nor could she communicate her thoughts and feelings. We have no way of knowing whether this is what Alberta would have wanted. We do know, however, that most people do not want to suffer, and that they do want to leave an inheritance for their children, grandchildren, nieces, and nephews.

Alberta's story is typical and quite common. As technology advances and as our senior population grows, millions of Americans will be facing similar circumstances.

It breaks my heart to share this story, but there are so many Alberta Coles out there, and I've taken care of more than I can count. Sadly, her story could have been even more graphic and painful than the way in which I've chosen to write it.

In the ER, when I examine a person who has long-standing mental and physical deterioration, and who lives in a nursing home, I have several competing reactions. Sometimes I just rationalize: this is the system, I'm part of it, and I do my job as best I can. At other times I get angry, because of the agony we put the patient through, and because of the time, energy, money, and medical talent spent on treatment that neither cures nor comforts. Third, I feel guilty, because I'm not taking steps to stop the process. Writing this book helps, but what will I do tomorrow if another Alberta is presented for my care? The best answer is for each of us to be sure that we don't end up in Alberta's situation.

# 4

## Step One

### Overview of the Forms

We can lick gravity, but sometimes the paperwork is overwhelming.

WERNER VON BRAUN

Let's take a look at how we can make medical care decisions for ourselves in situations and at times when it's difficult or impossible to make our wishes known.

Every state has a simple and legal way to do this, called an advance directive. There are some minor differences between states, so you should be sure to follow the rules in the state where you live. (These are outlined in the Resources section at the end of this book.)

To recap, there are four main parts of the advance directive package.

1. *Choosing the kind of care you want*: This is called a "Living Will," "Treatment Preferences," or "Instructions for Health Care."
2. *Choosing someone to act on your behalf when you cannot*: This is referred to as a "Medical Power of Attorney," with the person being called a "Health Care Agent."
3. *After-death instructions*: These include organ or body donation, disposition of the body, and funeral arrangements.
4. *Documentation*: This refers to the signatures and witnesses that make the advance directive legally enforceable.

Another well-known and highly regarded approach is called "Five Wishes." Their forms are available at 888-594-7437, www.agingwithdignity.org. The five wishes are as follows:

1. My wish for the person I want to make health care decisions for me when I can't make them.
2. My wish for the kind of medical treatment I want or don't want.
3. My wish for how comfortable I want to be.
4. My wish for how I want people to treat me.
5. My wish for what I want my loved ones to know.

Each of these wishes is followed by a list of options, all of which are written in simple, clear language. The approach is organized and complete. Still, each person needs to carefully reflect on their values and desires as they fill out the "Five Wishes" format.

Both the advance directive and the "Five Wishes" forms are only four to five pages long, with just a few choices to make. Checking or initialing a box answers most of the questions. While it usually takes time to think about these decisions, the forms themselves can be completed in only a few minutes.

Religious groups sometimes have their own preferred formats. For example, there is a Catholic advance health care directive. It is similar to non-Catholic advance directives, but the Catholic one includes statements such as: "In all circumstances, I oppose any act or omission that of itself or by intention will cause my death, even for the purpose of eliminating suffering. I direct that all decisions be made in accord with Catholic moral teachings as contained in such documents as the following: Pope John Paul II, *Care for Patients in a 'Permanent' Vegetative State* (March 20, 2004)" (excerpt from the Catholic Diocese of Wilmington, Delaware).

One Jewish approach to advance directives expresses Jewish values and states: "I want Jewish values and teachings to guide and inform the way I live through all times in my life, including times when I may be temporarily unable to communicate, am seriously ill, or in the final stages of my life."

It is also important to note that anyone can create his or her own advance directive. Any of these forms can be used as models. There is nothing that reduces the value of an advance directive written by an individual. It is just as legally binding as any other advance directive. An attorney is often consulted in these cases, to be sure that all the elements are covered and that nothing is left out.

Advance directives do not expire, but they can be changed at any time. A new advance directive automatically invalidates any prior ones.

These are important documents. As such, they should be reviewed periodically. They should also be stored in a safe place, with copies made available to your physician, your health care agent (the individual who holds your medical power of attorney), and key family members and friends. Since, by their nature, these documents only become operative when you are incapacitated, and occasionally under emergency conditions that require immediate decisions, it is critical that others know where they are and what they contain.

## 5

# Outlooks and Outcomes

The hardest thing to learn in life is which bridge to cross and
which to burn.

DAVID RUSSELL

Each of us has our own way of facing our end. Here are two
stories of men taking very different approaches.

Michael Simmons was a methodical and passionate man, with
four primary interests in life. One was his profession. He had always
known he wanted to be a doctor. After graduating from medical
school, he served in the Navy for two years during the Vietnam War,
and then completed his training in internal medicine. Michael was
a "doctor's doctor," setting aside time each day to study medical
journals and textbooks for his own continuing education, making
sure he was aware of all the latest scientific findings. He was also a
"patient's doctor": his devotion to his patients' care was what we'd
all like to receive from our physicians.

His second passion was his 25-foot Boston Whaler. He took
meticulous care of his craft, working on it every available weekend.
He kept careful maintenance records, as well as a log of every guest
and outing. He'd cruised from his home port down the Inland Passage to Florida. He attended boat shows to keep up on the latest
gear, and he wrote articles for boating magazines.

His third passion was staying fit. A varsity baseball player in
college, he'd always worked out and stayed in shape. He never
smoked, drank alcohol, or used any drugs. He was as straight-arrow
as anyone.

Last, and most important, Michael loved his family. His wife

Carla was his closest friend and companion. His daughter Rachel inherited his interest in science. She worked for a research company and was the mother of two young children.

Michael's symptoms began gradually and with great subtlety. At the start, he noticed that he seemed tired after what had previously been routine exertion. This didn't make any sense to him. He intensified his workout regimen, but the weakness and fatigue only got worse. He developed heartburn after eating, unusual in someone who had always been a robust eater and had no risk factors for acid reflux. His medical work-up was not revealing: routine tests were normal. Michael had access to the best medical specialists, and various theories were proposed. He eventually became convinced that his symptoms were due to the side effects of cholesterol-lowering drugs. He stopped the drugs, but the symptoms persisted.

Over the months, Michael's symptoms became more pronounced. At least one night a week he would be awakened from a sound sleep by choking spasms and have difficulty catching his breath. On two occasions he had to go to the emergency room before he could regain normal breathing. Michael had an inkling of what was causing his problem, but his suspicion was too horrifying even to share with Carla. More work-ups followed. Again all routine tests, including CT scans, were negative, but careful nerve and muscle tests showed deterioration. The diagnostic choices were limited, and as all other possible diseases were ruled out, only one remained. It was what Michael had feared: amyotrophic lateral sclerosis (ALS).

Commonly known as Lou Gehrig's disease, ALS is a progressive neuromuscular condition, starting in nerve cells in the spinal cord. As these cells die, the muscles they control fail. Eventually most patients are not able to stand or walk, get in or out of bed on their own, or use their hands and arms. In Michael's case, the nerve cells that were the first to go were in his throat, affecting his ability to swallow, chew, and speak. ALS does not affect cognitive function, so these patients are completely aware and mentally competent. There is no specific treatment, and average survival after diagnosis is three to five years. But for reasons no one understands, a small percentage of ALS patients live far longer—surviving 10 or even 20 or 30 years after diagnosis.

Michael observed his body's deterioration with scientific attention. He watched the fasciculations (the twitching of muscles in their death throes) that were visible through the skin in his forearms and legs. Michael had taken care of patients with ALS and seen them die. He knew what was in store for him: an inexorable downhill course culminating in death, possibly caused by an inability to breathe.

Almost immediately after this diagnosis, Michael made a decision that he would do nothing to prolong his life. For a time he contemplated suicide, but then rejected it as too upsetting for Carla and Rachel. Instead, Michael watched his body deteriorate, and he grew more and more despondent. He knew better than most that disease has nothing to do with fairness, but he still resented his fate. He was only 58 years old. He had always taken such good care of himself and tried so hard to do good for others.

Michael knew there were options to make his decline more comfortable and keep him functioning for the longest time possible. Physical therapy could help accommodate his bodily limitations. Speech therapy could help with his increasingly slurred speech. There were assistive devices to help with breathing and communication, and motorized wheelchairs to compensate for the growing deficits in his mobility. Carla urged him to make use of these aids, but Michael declined them all. His medical practice had already become limited to paperwork. Boating was out of the question. Driving, and even walking, grew progressively more difficult. Finally he put in for early retirement.

Carla tried to give Michael the best quality of life possible. She still prayed that he would be one of the lucky long-term survivors, but when she considered his situation realistically, she knew he didn't have much time left. Before he became too disabled, they managed a cruise to Alaska. Michael was in a wheelchair, and they couldn't participate in most of the shore excursions, but it gave him an opportunity to once again be on the water, with the sea he loved so much. At home, there were frequent visits from Rachel and the grandchildren, as well as from friends, colleagues, patients, and cousins who came from as far away as Europe to say their farewells.

Michael made a few concessions to prolonging his life. When he could no longer swallow comfortably without choking, he agreed to a gastrostomy tube. Now he took all hydration and nutrition directly into his stomach. When breathing became too difficult, he began using a positive-pressure ventilation device called a BiPAP to help move air in and out of his lungs.

His physicians urged him to have a tracheostomy, so that when the BiPAP no longer provided enough help, he would be able to transition to a full ventilator. They stressed that his mind was as sharp as ever, and that although a ventilator would prevent him from speaking, he could employ computers and other devices to communicate. There were still many avenues open to him for the enjoyment of life. They pointed to the example of Stephen Hawking, the world-renowned physicist who has survived over 30 years with ALS, continuing his distinguished scientific career despite being almost completely paralyzed and on a ventilator.

Michael's doctors and his friends respected his decision not to prolong his life, even if they couldn't really understand his reasoning. After all, while he was uncomfortable, he wasn't in pain. Why not keep going? Characteristically, Michael had based his decision on what to him was a rational assessment of his situation. If he couldn't do the things he loved—practice medicine, be on his boat, exercise vigorously, and spend active quality time with his family—then he didn't want to continue living. To him, these were the most important things in life, and without them, living had no purpose. This perspective was troubling to almost everyone, including Carla. But she and Michael had agreed that they would each honor the wishes of the other in sickness and in health.

As Michael grew weaker, he no longer left his house. He spent most days in bed, entertained by old movies on TV. For the last five months of his life, Michael needed virtually 24-hour care. This primarily fell on Carla until the last six weeks, when Rachel took family and medical leave from her job so she could move in with her parents. Friends and family pitched in to support Carla and Rachel with meals, errand running, and company.

A turning point came when hospice was consulted. This led to almost daily visits by the staff, something appreciated by both Michael and Carla. Hospice provided a number of important services. First, there were respite times for Carla and Rachel. Second, hospice taught them skills to help take care of Michael, making the daily chores of feeding, washing, and using the toilet easier and less taxing. Third, hospice provided a medication regimen that relieved some of Michael's worst symptoms. Michael frequently experienced the agony of "air hunger," the sensation of drowning caused by an inability to get enough air into his lungs. These episodes were treated by using medicines to reduce pain and anxiety, combined with suctioning his airway to clear out mucus. The team worked to balance Michael's medications, giving him enough morphine to keep the air hunger at bay, while not sedating him any more than was necessary.

Soon after his diagnosis, Michael had rewritten his advance directive to reflect his current thinking. He stated what he wanted and then put Carla in charge. As Michael withdrew, it became Carla's responsibility to handle all the medical decisions. This was hard, demanding, and stressful. They'd been married over 30 years, and she knew her husband better than anyone. She didn't want to lose him a minute sooner than necessary, but—tough as it was—she was determined to do what he had asked of her.

In his final days, Michael was awake for only brief periods. His pulse became rapid, his skin clammy, and his extremities cold. His breathing was labored, and, as the oxygen level in his blood fell, his mental functions began to deteriorate. Finally the oxygen dropped so low that his heart was unable to keep working, and, with a last gasp and shudder, he died in Carla's arms, 15 months after his diagnosis.

When Joseph Kranz's wife Edith died from a pulmonary embolism, the last thing she told him was not to mourn her too long. She said, "Life is a gift. Take all of it you can. Be there for the family."

Joseph and Edith had had a good life together. They'd been married for 50 years and had three children, now grown with families of their own. A first-generation child of German immigrants, Joseph was a self-made American success story. He worked hard and was always ready to make the most of his opportunities. He earned a degree in civil engineering, graduating in the early 1960s, just as construction was beginning on the national interstate highway system. He ended his career as the senior partner in a prosperous engineering firm, retiring when he turned 70.

He and Edith enjoyed another few years together before a broken hip led to the embolism that took her life. Joseph was deeply saddened, but he kept his perspective and took Edith's advice to heart. He stayed active and increased his charitable work, even endowing the Kranz Wing at their local hospital.

Joseph enjoyed fairly good health. He hadn't smoked in over 20 years and drank alcohol in moderation. He'd been diagnosed with high blood pressure at age 50, but the condition was controlled by medication. At age 80, he noticed that his legs seemed swollen, and he started having episodes of sweating at night. Then he found a small lump in his armpit. It didn't hurt, but it hadn't been there before. He could no longer ignore the symptoms.

Joseph was admitted to the hospital, where he underwent numerous tests and procedures: blood work, imaging scans, bone marrow analysis, a biopsy of lymph gland tissue with microscopic analysis, and consultations with various specialists. Finally his doctor had the diagnosis: lymphoma.

Lymphoma is a cancer of the immune-system cells called lymphocytes. There are many types of lymphoma, depending on the specific immune cells involved, but it was clear that Joseph's case was advanced.

Treatment of lymphoma is complicated, so Joseph was referred to an oncologist. Dr. Patel was guardedly optimistic. She told Joseph that most patients survive more than five years, but there was no way to predict what would happen in an individual case. Joseph might do well, but he already was older than most patients with lymphoma.

Prior to beginning chemotherapy, a catheter tube was placed in a large vein in Joseph's chest, creating a special opening (port) located just below the skin. A port can be used to infuse medications without having to find a new vein for each cycle of chemotherapy.

Dr. Patel explained that there would be several cycles of chemo, and that while the medications were balanced to reduce side effects, these were not completely avoidable. As predicted, Joseph's hair fell out, he felt sick and tired, and he had a sore mouth. His family helped him as best they could, and a day nurse was hired to take care of him during the week, when everyone was at work.

The experience shook Joseph. For the first time in his life, he was not in control. This brush with his own death frightened him, but it also energized him. He was a fighter; he wasn't going to let cancer get the better of him. He began to research his medical condition. He pored over the latest studies on lymphoma, its causes and treatments. He found inspiring stories of long-term survivors. He reviewed medical journals, and he began to contact national and international authorities about cutting-edge therapies. He read about alternative treatments, including vitamin and vaccine therapies. He even investigated cryonics, keeping people in a frozen state after death until a cure for their problem could be found, but he decided that this approach was not sufficiently developed—yet.

Dr. Patel suggested a consultation for Joseph with the palliative care program at the hospital. Recent studies had demonstrated that terminally ill patients who participated in a palliative care program, even while pursuing aggressive treatment, lived longer and had a better quality of life than those who waited till the end to get help for their symptoms. But Joseph was suspicious. Wasn't "palliative care" just another name for hospice? And wasn't hospice for those who had no chance of recovery? Dr. Patel tried to explain the distinctions, but Joseph wasn't buying it. "It sounds like giving up to me," he said. Joseph went through several rounds of therapy over the next four years. When one drug stopped working, Dr. Patel would try another. Joseph was ever hopeful for a new and better treatment, but eventually the lymphoma stopped responding.

When Joseph had completed his advance directive, he'd studied the forms carefully. In each case, he chose to prolong his life as long as possible. He didn't want "to pull the plug," because "who knows what treatment might be discovered tomorrow?" He didn't want to miss out on a miracle cure because he'd given up too soon.

Joseph designated his eldest son Gary as his health care agent. Gary and his siblings had conflicting emotions. On the one hand, they loved their father deeply, and they treasured these last four years that the chemo had bought them. But on the other hand, they could see the pain and suffering he endured with each round of treatment. Sometimes the cure seemed worse than the disease.

When Gary mentioned his concerns, Joseph was a little offended. Didn't Gary and the others want him to survive as long as there was a chance for a cure? Were they anxious to get their hands on his money sooner? Gary quickly backed off, assuring his father that he would abide by his wishes to the letter.

Joseph asked about getting a stem cell transplant, but Dr. Patel was skeptical. A transplant meant finding an acceptable donor, followed by intensive chemo and radiation therapy to wipe out the patient's bone marrow and immune system. Then the new bone marrow would be infused, and it could take weeks or months to gauge the response. During that time the patient would be in isolation, at risk from even the most minor illness or complication. At age 84, weakened by years of cancer therapy, Joseph would be unlikely to survive such an intense regimen.

But Joseph was adamant. He wanted this chance, and he was willing to pay for it, even if his insurance wouldn't cover the bill. He called the hospital's administrator and reminded him of his donations to the institution.

Gary and the family were shocked that Joseph was willing to try a difficult experimental treatment that, at best, might buy him only a few more months of life. Wouldn't it be better for him to die at home or in a hospice, rather than in the hospital, undergoing uncomfortable procedures? But they had learned not to question their father's wishes. In his darker moments, Gary wondered if his father's dogged fight for life came from his will to live or from his fear of death.

As Joseph went through the preparations for a bone marrow transplant, his condition grew worse. It got harder and harder for him to breathe, and a fever set in. He called Gary to take him to the ER, where pneumonia, kidney failure, and low blood counts were diagnosed. In critical condition, Joseph was admitted to the intensive care unit. Within a few hours, his blood pressure began to fall as sepsis (widespread bloodstream infection) developed. Infusions to boost his blood pressure were given.

By the time the rest of the family arrived, Joseph had lapsed into a coma, his breathing maintained by a ventilator. Dr. Patel met with the family, explaining that the sepsis was not responding to treatment: Joseph's immune system was too battered. Their father would not regain consciousness, nor recover sufficiently to undergo the transplant. She advised them to say their goodbyes and remove the ventilator.

Gary's younger siblings wanted to follow the doctor's advice. They felt their father had suffered enough. He had fought the good fight, but now it was time to go. Gary hesitated. They gathered at Joseph's bedside in the ICU cubicle, finding space to stand between the machines and the monitors. Joseph burned with fever, yet his hands were cold and darkening, showing signs of necrosis (tissue death). But Gary had promised not to "pull the plug." They took turns keeping their ICU vigil until the next afternoon, when the sepsis overwhelmed him and Joseph's heart stopped beating.

Both of these men made decisions that I would not have. If I had ALS, was not in pain, and my mental functions were intact, I believe I'd choose to keep going as long as possible with a tracheotomy, breathing assistance, and every modern device to help me move about and communicate. If I had advanced lymphoma, I'd take a shot or two at chemo, but then I'd go home and allow nature to take its course, after making sure I would be kept as comfortable as possible for as long as possible. I've seen patients die of advanced sepsis, and it's not a good death.

In both of these stories, the family would have made a different choice than that of their dying loved one. But the decision belongs to the person involved, not to his or her family. As a physician, my job is to provide the best information possible, without partiality or prejudice. As a legislator, I want to ensure that everyone is empowered to make these decisions without undue outside interference. Even if I disagree with a decision a patient has made, I try not to question or judge, and I carry out that person's advance directive as closely as possible.

# 6

## Step Two

### *Choosing the Kind of Care You Want*

Because I could not stop for Death, he kindly stopped for me—
the carriage held but just Ourselves—and Immortality.

EMILY DICKINSON

The first section of an advance directive goes by different names.
It might be called a "Living Will," "Treatment Preferences," or "Instructions for Health Care." But all these terms apply to the same
thing, so, for the sake of clarity, I'll refer to this component as a living will. It addresses the following question: What are the basic
values and standards you'd like to see applied should you be unable
to make decisions for yourself?

A living will gives guidance to physicians and families as they
make determinations about the kind of care the person wants. The
advantage of a living will is that it allows people to outline the type
of care that they feel is appropriate for them. The limitation of a living will is that it's difficult to anticipate every complexity of specific
medical decision making that may arise. For example, the living will
may say, "Keep me comfortable and pain free." But sometimes it can
be hard to translate what is "comfortable" and "pain free" into appropriate dosages of sedatives or narcotics. That's why living wills
work best when the person has also designated a health care agent
who holds their medical power of attorney (more about this later).

Some living will forms include a statement of values. This is the
opportunity to offer, in a few sentences of your own composition,
something about your goals and wishes during the last part of your
life.

For example, one person might say: "To me, the life of the mind is the most important thing. If it appears that my mind is not functioning, if I'm not aware of what's going on around me, with no chance of recovery, if I can't relate to people who are around me, then I don't consider it worthwhile to prolong my life. Just keep me comfortable and pain free, and let nature take its course."

Another example might be: "I believe in the wholeness of life. Even if I don't appear to be able to comprehend what's going on around me, there still could be consciousness and awareness within me. My experience, however it may appear to others, is still my experience, and I value it. Plus, there have been cases of people who seemed to be in a coma who recovered. So please keep me alive as long as possible."

Following this statement of values, the next section involves details about specific care situations. This is the most important aspect of a living will. Typically, these choices come in three categories: do little or nothing, do something, or do everything.

Here's an example from Maryland's "Treatment Preference" section:

Preference in case of terminal condition.
If my doctors certify that my death from a terminal condition is imminent, even if life-sustaining procedures are used:
    1. Keep me comfortable and allow natural death to occur. I do not want any medical interventions used to try to extend my life. I do not want to receive nutrition and fluids by tube or other medical means.
    OR
    2. Keep me comfortable and allow natural death to occur. I do not want medical interventions used to try to extend my life. If I am unable to take enough nourishment by mouth, however, I want to receive nutrition and fluids by tube or other means.
    OR
    3. Try to extend my life for as long as possible, using all available interventions that in reasonable medical judgment

would prevent or delay my death. If I am unable to take enough nourishment by mouth, I want to receive nutrition and fluids by tube or other medical means.

The California form approaches this slightly differently, in a section called "End-of-Life Decisions":

I direct that my health care providers and others involved in my care provide, withhold, or withdraw treatment in accordance with the choice I have marked below:
Choice Not To Prolong Life:
_____ I do not want my life to be prolonged if (1) I have an incurable and irreversible condition that will result in my death within a relatively short time, (2) I become unconscious and, to a reasonable degree of medical certainty, I will not regain consciousness, or (3) the likely risks and benefits of treatment would outweigh the expected benefits.
OR
Choice To Prolong Life:
_____ I want my life prolonged as long as possible within the limits of generally accepted health care standards.

It should be clear that an advance directive does not in any way limit care. It merely defines the type and degree of care that a person wants. How one answers these questions is entirely personal. The choices made should stem from an individual's understanding of life and its meaning. Let's now talk about a few of the specifics.

## Hydration and Nourishment

As the dying process sets in, appetite dwindles. In fact, many experts look at appetite loss in a severely ill person as one of the signs that the end is near. Eating and drinking are basic human activities, surpassed only by breathing as a necessity for life. As the body begins to shut down, the demand for nourishment fades. The body quiets, metabolism slows, and the desire to eat and drink recedes.

Sometimes patients only want enough water to keep their lips and mouth moist.

Debates surround the issue of whether withholding nourishment is painful for a person dying of other medical causes, and therefore whether or not it is ethical. This is a complex topic, and there is a spectrum of opinions. Often what to do depends on the specifics of each case.

Let's take the example of a person dying of cancer. He or she has had all possible treatments, but the cancer has spread throughout the person's body. Appetite is gone, and the individual has lost weight, becoming skeletal. There is pain, but it is well controlled with pain medicine. The person is getting weaker every day, with only limited periods of being awake and aware. Breathing is labored, and the individual is bed-bound. In this case, trying to extend life with fluids is useless and in fact may prolong the agony.

Or consider a young man or woman who has suffered a severe traumatic brain injury. Such a person is comatose: an electroencephalogram (EEG) is a flat line, and a brain CT scan shows that the brain tissue has deteriorated and been replaced by fluid. There is no hope of improvement or recovery. However, the rest of the patient's bodily functions work normally. The person breathes, the heart pumps blood, and the digestive tract can process food. The patient requires constant monitoring and hourly care, turning to avoid skin sores, and physical therapy to minimize limb contractures. In this case, nutrition can prolong the individual's life, sometimes for years. Whether this should be done or not is something that is difficult to decide. If the patient has an advance directive and chose one of the options mentioned above, then the caregivers would know what to do. If the patient had designated a health care agent, then that person could decide. But if nothing had been written and no one designated as an agent, then choosing the proper course of action is problematic.

Here's a third case. The patient has an injury high on the spinal cord, resulting in paralysis from the neck down. Unable to move anything below the neck, this person requires daily care for all physical needs. But the patient is awake, alert, conscious, oriented, and can communicate. This individual falls into the category of having an end-stage condition, which is defined as a condition that continues in its course until death, and one that already has resulted in loss of capacity and complete physical dependency. In this case, since the patient can make his or her wishes known, a living will would not be triggered. Such a patient's choice of whether or not to receive nutrition becomes like any other adult's choice of whether or not to eat. It is rare for such patients to choose to refuse sustenance, but the law protects their right to do so without being subjected to forced feedings.

## Pain Management

No one wants to suffer needlessly, and modern medicines and pain management techniques have made tremendous progress in relieving pain and discomfort. Still, there are issues to be considered.

Some pain medicines can hasten death. For example, narcotics such as morphine, Dilaudid, codeine, and OxyContin are mainstays of pain treatment. But these medicines have side effects, including respiratory depression—reducing the person's ability to breathe. An overdose can lead to death. But it's a fine line in distinguishing when pain relief crosses over to actually speeding the death process along. When does effective pain relief become assisted suicide, which is often a felony? The state has an interest in protecting its citizens' lives, but laws can also have a chilling effect on caregivers. If it were perceived that a doctor "overprescribed" narcotics for pain, even at the request of a patient, then that doctor could face criminal or civil prosecution.

Nonetheless, pain can and should be treated. There have been unfortunate instances of narcotics being withheld due to fear of creating an addiction, even when the potential "addict" has only weeks to live. Many patients have told me that it is not death they fear, but the pain that might go along with the dying process. Physicians and patients should keep open a dialogue about the best ways to reduce and relieve pain. As the patient's condition changes, so might their choices.

## CPR

Another key decision is whether or not you want cardio-pulmonary resuscitation. Most people know the basics of CPR. It's been popularized on TV and in movies, as well as in first aid courses. In its simplest form, the victim receives airway clearing, mouth-to-mouth breathing, and chest compressions. Sometimes an automated external defibrillator (AED) can be used. AEDs are often found in public places, such as airports, large buildings, and arenas. Using computerized programs, AEDs shock the patient's heart and, it is hoped, restore a normal heart rhythm.

The most sophisticated forms of CPR are provided in hospitals by medical staff, or by full-level paramedics in the field. In these cases, the patient may be intubated (a plastic tube inserted into the airway) and get medications such as epinephrine, lidocaine, and atropine by vein. In hospitals these CPR events are called "codes," and one might hear the words "code blue, CCU" over a hospital's public address system. A code can last 5 minutes to an hour, depending on the patient's response to treatment and other factors.

There are dramatic occurrences of recovery after CPR, but, unfortunately, despite years of research and study, CPR is still rarely effective. Survival rates from CPR started in a community setting range from about 4 percent to 6 percent. These rates are somewhat higher in hospitals, but not dramatically so. A few years back, an article in the *New England Journal of Medicine* compared CPR success rates on television shows like *ER* and *Chicago Hope* with real world statistics. Perhaps not surprisingly, George Clooney and his colleagues saved more than 75 percent of their patients. I only wish we could match that record.

The biggest factors in CPR success are the previous health of the victim, the time elapsed between the cardiac arrest and CPR, the technique used by the person performing CPR, and the underlying cause of the arrest. For example, a drowning victim who's promptly pulled from a cold lake has a better chance of successfully being revived than the elderly and debilitated victim of a blocked coronary artery.

As we saw, Alberta Cole's lack of an advance directive meant that doctors performed multiple medical interventions on her. Whether these helped or hurt; whether she would have wanted them or not; whether the extra months of life battling bedsores, bladder infections, broken ribs, and dementia justified the pain she endured; and whether the expense was really needed are all questions that can never be answered. Nor could her family or doctors confidently make a decision not to perform those interventions, especially because there was a difference of opinion among her children.

# 7

## Karen Quinlan, Nancy Cruzan, and Terri Schiavo

### It's Not Just about Older People

Live as if you were to die tomorrow. Learn as if you were to live forever.

GANDHI

We tend to think about end-of-life questions in the context of the elderly and the chronically ill, but the three most famous U.S. legal cases on this issue all involved healthy young women. While most Americans are familiar with the case of Theresa Marie (Terri) Schiavo, whose "right to die" dominated headlines and national debate in 2004 and 2005, the two landmark cases on this issue came much earlier.

These three cases were all instrumental in changing attitudes, public opinion, and, ultimately, laws.

As you read these tragic stories of family heartbreak, extensive medical treatments, and years-long legal wrangling, consider how they would be managed today if each of these three unfortunate women had completed an advance directive beforehand. The circumstances clearly demonstrate that advance directives are for everyone of adult age. Of course, how one completes an advance directive will change from age 18 to 28 to 58 to 88, which is why these documents need to be updated periodically.

## Karen Ann Quinlan

Thirty-five years ago Karen Ann Quinlan was the center of what became the first major case on the complex legal issues regarding the right to die. The New Jersey Supreme Court characterized the case as a "matter of transcendent importance," because it raised two fundamental questions: (1) is there a right to refuse life-saving medical treatment, and (2) when, if ever, can a guardian exercise that right on behalf of an incompetent patient (someone unable to make decisions for himself or herself).

Despite extensive testing, no cause was ever determined for 21-year-old Karen Ann Quinlan's collapse on April 15, 1975. Unable to breathe on her own, Karen was placed on a respirator. As the months rolled by, she remained in a vegetative state with no higher brain activity. While the experts agreed that her chances for a return to any kind of functioning were remote, Karen Quinlan was not considered brain dead. As a result, her attending physicians, as well as the medical experts who testified at trial, concluded that to remove Karen from the respirator would both deviate from the standard practice of medicine and be tantamount to a homicide and an act of euthanasia.

At that time, medical science was just beginning to evolve, so that patients who had previously died of illnesses like Karen's were surviving. But definitions of "brain death," "vegetative state," and "incompetent to make a decision" were still not well worked out.

At the beginning of the ordeal, Karen's parents authorized her treating physician to do everything within his power to keep their daughter alive, believing that she might recover. As their hope faded that Karen would regain mental functions, Mr. and Mrs. Quinlan sought the advice of their parish priest. He advised them that given Karen's circumstances, the termination of life-support would be a permissible practice according to the teachings of the Roman Catholic Church. The Quinlans asked the hospital to discontinue all extraordinary measures to keep Karen alive, including the use of a respirator. They released the physicians and the hospital from any and all liability in connection with their actions. But even with the authorization and release, neither Karen's treating physician nor the hospital would agree to terminate the use of the respirator.

In 1975 it would have been highly unusual for a 21-year-old to provide any instruction to her parents and physicians in the event she should become unable to manage her own care. Indeed, at that time very few legal and medical professionals had any concept of the notion of an advance directive or living will, and such documents were virtually unknown to individuals who were not involved in medicine or law.

In response to seeing the deaths of family members and relatives of close friends, Karen was quoted by her mother, her sister, and a friend as having made statements to the effect that she would never want to be kept alive by extraordinary means. Mrs. Quinlan testified that Karen "was very full of life . . . and did not want to be kept alive in any way where she would not enjoy life to the fullest."

Given this evidence, Mr. Quinlan petitioned the New Jersey courts to appoint him legal guardian of Karen's person and property and to "intervene in the best interests of Karen Quinlan and allow her to die a natural death."

The lower court ruled against Mr. Quinlan by holding that Karen's right to privacy, claimed on her behalf by her father, was trumped by both the medical professional's duty to provide life-sustaining treatment, and the judicial obligation to choose continued life over death. Thus the court found that there is no constitutional right to die that could be offered by a parent for an incompetent adult child.

Mr. Quinlan appealed to the New Jersey Supreme Court. That court overturned the lower court's ruling and gave Mr. Quinlan the right to authorize the removal of the respirator. It held that the constitutional right to privacy was broad enough to include an individual's decision to refuse medical treatment under certain circumstances. The court found that had Karen been able to make decisions for herself, she would have chosen to discontinue the use of the respirator, even if that decision would have resulted in her death. The court also said that Karen's individual rights had overcome the interest of the State, and thus she had a right to die.

The *Quinlan* case was important for recognizing that the right to withdraw medical treatment is protected by the Constitution and that a designated guardian could make medical decisions for an incompetent patient. This was a remarkable shift away from the paternalism prevalent in the medical profession at the time, and it marked another step in the trend toward patient autonomy.

The *Quinlan* case also recognized that the decision to withdraw life-sustaining treatment depends not only on whether a patient's existence may be prolonged, but also on the quality of life the patient might reasonably expect.

The Quinlans won for their daughter the right to die "with grace and dignity," and she was weaned from the respirator in March 1976. Karen continued to breathe on her own, and her parents chose to continue artificial feeding. Karen lived for nine more years, until 1985, when she died at age 31 of respiratory failure brought on by pneumonia.

It was becoming clear that advances in medical care were raising complex issues. People could have their bodily functions sustained almost indefinitely, even if they couldn't think, move, or act for themselves. Who would make the decisions about their care, and on what basis would those decisions be made? The *Quinlan* case was the first major case to bring these issues to the fore.

## Nancy Beth Cruzan

Nancy Cruzan was 25 years old when, on the night of January 11, 1983, she was involved in a single-car accident in Jasper County, Missouri. Nancy was thrown from her overturned vehicle and found lying face-down in a ditch without detectable breathing or heartbeat. Although she never regained consciousness, paramedics at the scene were able to restart her breathing with a tube, and her heart began to beat again after stimulation with medication. At the hospital she was found to have severe brain injury, complicated by a long period without oxygen. Permanent brain damage results after 6 minutes of oxygen deprivation, and experts estimated that Nancy had been deprived of oxygen for a period of at least 12 to 14 minutes.

Nancy remained in a coma, with no signs of higher brain function. Although she could breathe on her own, she could not swallow, so nutrition and hydration were provided by a gastrostomy feeding tube. Despite intense therapy and rehabilitation over the following weeks, Nancy's condition did not improve. She was transferred from the rehabilitation facility to her home, where she was cared for by her family and round-the-clock nurses. After developing pneumonia, Nancy was admitted to the Mt. Vernon State Hospital on October 19, 1983, where she remained in a persistent vegetative state.

Nancy's parents, Lester and Joyce Cruzan, had been appointed her coguardians and conservators. In 1988, after four years without improvement in their daughter's condition, the Cruzans asked the court for permission to stop artificial feeding and hydration. At the trial, the court heard extensive testimony from physicians and nurses, and it concluded that Nancy had lost all higher cognitive brain function, as well as the ability to swallow food and water, and that this condition was irreversible.

The trial court further found that Nancy had said, in a conversation with her housemate, that she did not want to be kept alive by artificial means if she could not live "halfway normally." The court concluded that to deny Nancy's parents the authority to act under these circumstances would be to deprive Nancy of equal protection under the law. The court ordered the state hospital employees to carry out the wishes of Nancy's parents and withdraw her feeding tube. In part because this was a case without precedent, Nancy's court-appointed guardian appealed the decision.

The Missouri Supreme Court overturned the lower court, ruling that there was neither a constitutionally protected right to die nor sufficiently clear and convincing evidence that Nancy Cruzan would not wish to continue her vegetative existence. The majority further found that her parents, as guardians, had no right to make decisions on their daughter's behalf. Cruzan's parents appealed the Missouri decision, and in December 1989 the U.S. Supreme Court heard its first case concerning the right to die.

The *Cruzan* decision overturned the previous *Quinlan* case in that the Supreme Court held that any right to refuse treatment had to be balanced against a state's legitimate interest in maintaining life. Second, the majority rejected the idea that a person's quality of life should be considered in deciding to terminate life-sustaining treatment. Third, the court decided that statements made by Nancy Cruzan to her housemate did not meet the "clear and convincing" standard of proof required by Missouri law.

However, Justice Sandra Day O'Connor, while voting with the majority, took a different approach. She made it clear that the court's decision was to be applied only to the Missouri statute. She wrote that "the Court does not today decide the issue whether a State must also give effect to the decisions of a surrogate decision-maker." This meant that other states would have to resolve the matter for themselves.

Justice O'Connor's opinion motivated both the federal and state governments to enact or clarify living will and advance directive laws. In 1991 the Patient Self-Determination Act was passed by Congress and signed into law by President George H. W. Bush. All 50 states and the District of Columbia followed with laws of their own.

Two months after the Supreme Court's decision was issued, Nancy's parents asked the state court to consider new evidence from several of their daughter's coworkers. The coworkers testified that Nancy had said she would not want to live "like a vegetable." The judge ruled that these statements provided clear and convincing evidence of Nancy's intentions and ordered the hospital to comply with the request of Nancy's parents to have her feeding tube removed. This was done on December 14, 1990, and Nancy Cruzan died twelve days later, at the age of 33, surrounded by her family— six months after the Supreme Court's ruling, and almost eight years after the accident.

## Theresa Marie Schiavo

The case of another young woman, Terri Schiavo, became a contentious issue in the debate over the right to die and the right to privacy. Ultimately the case involved advocacy groups on all sides, as well as the president, Congress, and even the Vatican. Six times over the course of the case, the U.S. Supreme Court was asked to rule, and each time it declined to do so.

Terri Schiavo had been living in a persistent vegetative state since a cardiac arrest in 1990. In 1998, after many years of failed attempts to restore her brain function, Terri's husband Michael, as her guardian, asked that artificial feeding be stopped "so that she would die a natural death." He said that this was her stated preference should she ever become incapacitated with no hope of meaningful recovery. Terri's parents disagreed, arguing that their daughter was not in a persistent vegetative state, and that even if she were, she would not have wanted to have artificial life-support removed.

Beginning with a trial in the Florida courts, the issues were litigated, appealed, and relitigated. Terri's feeding tube was removed for the first time in 2001, but then was reinserted two days later, pending an appeal by her parents. The appeal was rejected, and the tube was removed again in 2003. Within six days the Florida legislature and Governor Jeb Bush enacted "Terri's Law," mandating the tube's reinsertion. Subsequently, Terri's Law was declared unconstitutional by the courts, and on March 18, 2005, Terri Schiavo's feeding tube was removed for the third and final time.

In the meantime, a media frenzy began. The Schiavo case was the number-one topic on the 24-hour news cycle, on talk shows, and at kitchen tables around the country.

Two days later, on March 20, Congress passed emergency legislation (the "Palm Sunday Compromise") to allow Terri's parents to petition the federal courts for the feeding tube to be reinserted. President George W. Bush flew back to Washington, D.C., from his vacation in Texas to sign the bill, and Terri's parents immediately followed up with a petition for an injunction in the Federal District Court. Arguments were heard the following day, after which the judge declined to order the reinsertion.

The next day, the 11th Circuit Court of Appeals in Atlanta upheld the Federal District Court's ruling, and one day later the U.S. Supreme Court once again refused to hear the case. This effectively ended all further appeals. Terri Schiavo died on March 31, 2005, with Michael at her side. An autopsy revealed extensive and irreversible brain damage.

One thing was clear from the beginning: had Terri Schiavo completed an advance directive, her wishes would have been known, and the firestorm of family, legal, and political conflict would have been avoided.

The chapter title says it all: "It's Not Just about Older People." The legal and medical circumstances of Quinlan, Cruzan, and Schiavo still apply to any of us. Every time I speak publicly about the need for advance directives, I get a range of reactions from audience members. "Why do I need one of those? I'm in good health." "This is for grandma and grandpa, not me." "This makes me sad. I'd rather not think about it."

Older people have more life experience to help them make the choices required by an advance directive. They are also more likely to need them before a younger person would. But young people can meet with catastrophes as well. Advance directives are about being prepared, about taking steps to spare others unnecessary heartache. Everyone should complete one, and there's no excuse not to.

# 8

## Dave Eckhart
### Who's in Charge?

A dying man needs to die, as a sleepy man needs to sleep, and
there comes a time when it is wrong, as well as useless, to resist.

STEWART ALSOP

Dave Eckhart was 72 years old and had been in excellent health
when he suddenly developed a severe headache, followed by slurred
speech and paralysis of his left arm and leg.

Dave was a businessman. He owned a small liquor store spe-
cializing in fine wines. His daughter Nancy had taken over the enterprise and ran it on a day-to-day basis, but Dave still enjoyed
coming to the store. He would show up two or three days per week.
Many of the customers were regulars, and Dave liked socializing
with them.

Dave's wife Ellen was also an active businessperson. She ran a
real estate firm. At age 70, she was fit and trim. She managed the
office and handled some sales calls and open houses, although she
left most of those to the younger sales force. Ellen had years of experience and valuable tips on how to close deals.

Their other child, Frank, had moved to Washington, D.C. He
was an attorney with the federal government and had a wife and
children. Family visits were frequent, and Dave and Ellen often took
care of their grandkids so Frank and his wife and Nancy and her
husband could have time on their own.

Dave was upstairs in the bathroom early Saturday morning
when the symptoms struck. Ellen was downstairs, but she heard
Dave groan and then slump to the floor. She ran upstairs and found

him. With difficulty Ellen helped Dave move to the bed. He was conscious, though frightened, and he could still move one side of his body. Ellen called 911, then Frank and Nancy, and waited for the paramedics.

In 8 minutes the paramedics arrived. Dave's condition hadn't changed. The paramedics started an IV, put on a cardiac monitor, and checked Dave's blood sugar, all while getting a brief medical history. Sometimes low blood sugar can mimic a stroke, and, if that's the case, the symptoms can be reversed quickly with intravenous glucose. But Dave was not a diabetic, and his sugar level was normal. So was his heart rhythm. The paramedics brought in a stretcher and called in to the hospital. They informed the emergency room nurse and doctor that they were bringing in a possible stroke victim.

Stroke is a general term that means that some part of the brain isn't getting an adequate blood supply. The region of the brain thus deprived fails to control the part of the nervous system that it is responsible for. So a stroke in the speech center will cause loss of speech, or one controlling movement in a leg will paralyze that limb.

Loss of blood supply can happen for several reasons. The most common is a blocked artery, usually due to atherosclerosis, or cholesterol build up. Like an old pipe, the artery gradually narrows, so that flow is reduced to a trickle and then blocked altogether. But stroke can also be due to bleeding inside the brain. A blood vessel can burst, both interrupting its blood delivery and causing swelling that cuts off the flow of other nearby vessels. Or a bit of blood clot or tissue from another part of the body, usually the heart, can break off and travel in the blood vessel until the channel becomes so small that it can't pass any farther. This is called an embolus. It then blocks blood flow in the vessel. Even a brain tumor can look like a stroke when symptoms start. The pressure of the tumor mass can also limit blood flow to a part of the brain.

A patient with a stroke from any of these causes can look exactly the same to the ER doctor. While there may be differences in the patient's history and ER exam that suggest one cause or another, the best quick test to find out what's happening is to get a CT scan of the head. The scan can show blocked blood flow, bleeding, or a tumor. Each of these has very different treatments, so a timely diagnosis is critical. For example, a blood vessel blocked by a blood clot might be treated with medications that dissolve clots. However, it would be disastrous to give that medication to someone who's bleeding and needs clots to form to stop the bleeding.

When Dave got to the ER, the staff, having been alerted by the paramedics, was ready. Blood was drawn, an intravenous line was established, and a neurologist was summoned. If Dave's stroke were the result of a blood clot (the most common scenario), a neurologist would be needed to manage the complex medical treatment that would ensue.

Dave's condition was changing for the worse. His level of consciousness was decreasing, and he was slipping into a coma. In order to protect his airway and to make sure his breathing continued, the ER doctor intubated him.

Dave was taken to the CT scanning room with Ellen and a nurse at his side. The CT scan took 10 minutes, and the on-call radiologist only needed to glance at the film to see what was going on. He called the ER doctor: "Mr. Eckhart has a massive intracranial hemorrhage. The bleeding is causing herniation." What this means is that the bleeding was so substantial that it was literally compressing the entire brain. Parts of Dave's brain were being shoved past their normal boundaries and down into his spinal canal.

The ER doctor immediately notified the neurosurgeon on call, as well as Dave's regular family doctor. He also took Dave's family to a private room to review the situation with them. Just as this discussion began, the ER doctor was pulled from the room because Dave's condition took a sudden downturn. He had a small seizure, and then he began what's known as decerebrate posturing. Dave's arms and legs became rigidly extended, his back and head arched, and his toes pointed down. This was a very bad sign, indicating severe, irreversible brain damage.

It had only been 1 hour since Dave fell in the bedroom at his home.

The neurosurgeon arrived, having already reviewed the CT scan. He and the ER doctor met with the family, and they described Dave's circumstances: "Mr. Eckhart has had a massive brain hemorrhage. The bleeding is deep inside the brain. The parts of his brain not directly injured have been under tremendous pressure from the expanding bleeding, and now they are impaired as well. It only takes a few minutes of oxygen deprivation to cause irreversible brain damage."

Ellen asked, "Can't you operate and stop the bleeding?"

The neurosurgeon answered: "Of course we can always operate, but this would be major surgery, and it's very unlikely he would survive. And even surgery will not restore him. It might keep him alive a few hours or a few days. Because he's in good health otherwise, he might survive for as much as a week. At this point he's breathing only because a respirator is breathing for him. His heart is strong and will keep beating, but his brain is dead. We're sorry, but there's nothing we can do. I wish there were, but realistically there isn't. You need some time alone to think about this."

Ellen, Frank, and Nancy struggled to take it all in. The shock was tremendous. Only an hour ago Dave was planning his day, full of activities. Now he was on a stretcher, effectively dead, his mind gone, his body living on.

The family went to the emergency room to be with their husband and father. They could see with their own eyes that Dave's body wasn't working. The respirator hummed, moving the air in and out of Dave's lungs. They held his hand and spoke quietly of their love and affection. They asked the ER doctor and nurse what was next. Dave would stay in the ER 2 to 3 more hours until a hospital bed was ready, and they could stay with him. But the staff said that the family ought to discuss what they wanted or what they thought Dave would want. Ellen knew that she and Dave had completed advance directives years ago. They were at home in a file cabinet. Frank went there to get Dave's.

Ellen recalled that Dave had served in the Army in Korea. He had seen death, and he had seen men with terrible head injuries. He'd seen men who'd lost their ability to function and to think. Dave thrived on his independence, and he'd often said that he never wanted to burden his family.

When Frank returned, they read Dave's advance directive. In it, he wrote that he did not want to be kept alive if he had no chance of recovery or if he had no chance of conscious life. He would want pain relief, but he would choose to allow nature to take its course. He did not want to be kept alive indefinitely by artificial means. He had designated Ellen as his health care agent.

The family discussed Dave's wishes and the circumstances he was in. They asked the ER doctor to return. What would happen if Dave were admitted and kept on a respirator? "Our best guess is that he could live for weeks or months, possibly even years. He would require constant care: feeding through tubes, complete personal hygiene. But he will not awaken, he will not talk, and he will not be aware of what's going on."

What if the respirator was stopped and the breathing tube pulled out? "He would likely stop breathing in a few minutes or hours. He would die, although sometimes patients like him may last longer. There is no way to know for sure."

But aren't there people who are in a coma for years and then wake up? "There have a been a few recorded cases, but even then, the recovery has been minimal. These rare cases have also been in younger people who suffered other kinds of brain injury, not the massive bleeding that is happening with Mr. Eckhart, where just about all the neurons in the brain are seriously damaged or dead."

Dave's advance directive also noted that he wanted to be an organ donor. A kidney transplant had saved a friend's child, and this had inspired Dave. The family wanted to honor Dave's wishes, and the Donate Life organization was contacted. A Donate Life counselor came to the hospital and joined the family. Questions were asked and answered. Was Dave too old to donate? No, age was not a problem. Dave's organs and body were in excellent shape, and everything would be closely examined before any transplantations were done. Would there be a cost? No cost to the family. Could they find out how Dave's organs were used? Yes, but only in general. Later, if the recipient agreed, contact information could be exchanged. When would the organs be removed? A team would be brought in to collect the organs at the moment Dave died.

Ellen, Frank, and Nancy notified their extended family: the grandkids who ranged in age from 7 to 16, close family friends, and relatives. Their minister was called and joined them at the hospital. Over the next few hours, the family grieved over what had befallen their loved one, but there were also lighter moments, recalling many aspects of Dave's life. Dave was never left alone, as family members went in and out of the room, keeping constant vigil. A few hours passed, and the central question remained: What would Dave want now?

Eventually Ellen was able to come to a decision. "Dave and I have had a wonderful life. We've done everything we could hope to do: family, career, travel, and time together. But Dave and I decided long ago that we would respect each other's wishes when the end was near. Now it's that time for Dave. I know what he would want. He told us, and he wrote it down. Dave would not want to go on like he is now. He'd want us to remember him as we knew him: father, friend, and member of the community. Let's all say good-bye. Then, let's bring the ER doctor back and ask him to pull the tube out and keep Dave comfortable until the end."

Dave died a few hours later. His organs were collected, and his gift saved three lives.

In 2008, I was the lead sponsor of a bill (House Bill 906) that simplified the process of organ donation in Maryland. Working on that bill allowed me to meet many people who received organs and the family members of those who had donated. Some people wept openly at the bill hearing, and I was deeply moved by their stories. Thanks to modern medical science, organ donation helped both the family of the donor and the recipient get through a very difficult time.

A dear friend was the mother of a 19-year-old man who died in a sudden, tragic accident. She spoke at her son's memorial service.

Others had preceded her and told stories of his life, but she spoke briefly to share the following: "When David was 16 and got his driver's license, he had no hesitation in designating himself as an organ donor. Today I received a letter that two people can now see because of corneal transplants, and 50 more are helped by his skin, bones, and tendons. And there are others whose lives were saved by his heart, lungs, pancreas, liver, and kidneys. Yes, he is gone, but not only does his memory live on, it gives us great comfort to know that the gift of his body continues and gives life to others."

# 9

# Step Three

## *Selecting Your Health Care Agent*

To be trusted is a greater compliment than being loved.

GEORGE MACDONALD

One of the most important parts of completing an advance directive is choosing the person who will be given your medical power of attorney. Designating someone to hold your medical power of attorney authorizes that individual to act as your health care agent.

Should you ever be in a situation where you cannot make medical decisions for yourself, your health care agent will be able to make those decisions for you. Obviously the person you select should be someone you know and trust. Ideally, you will discuss your wishes with a potential health care agent prior to any serious illness. A living will, wherein you choose the kind of care you want, can also be used as a guide for your health care agent.

What happens if you don't authorize a health care agent? Then decisions will be made for the medically ill person by a substitute, known as a surrogate. In most states there is an order of priority that is followed in selecting a surrogate. Typically the order is court-appointed guardian, spouse, adult child, parent, adult sibling, close friend or relative. However, it is easy to see how failing to name a health care agent can lead to problems. For example, what if two adult children disagree about the care of a parent? Or what happens when two siblings want different treatments for their brother? When this occurs, emotions run high and conflicts can escalate. Sometimes questions of money and potential inheritance issues cloud the medical decision-making process. Families can and do end up in court.

As stated above, a living will should be a guide for a health care agent. However, many medical decisions do not fall into easily recognizable categories. Should pneumonia be treated with antibiotics? Is an MRI really needed to evaluate a change in mental status? Is it time to discharge the patient from the hospital to a long-term care facility?

Designating a health care agent is one of the most important end-of-life care decisions one can make. So, who should be chosen?

Most people choose a spouse or another family member. However, a health care agent does not have to be a family member. It can be a close friend or other adviser. It's also important to designate a back-up health care agent or two in case the first-choice person isn't available. The names and contact information for the primary health care agent and the back-ups will be filled out on the advance directive form. If there is someone you specifically do not want involved in making your health care decisions, you can spell that out as well in your advance directive.

You can give other rights to your health care agent. For example, one form requests that the health care agent be allowed to ride in the ambulance with the patient and be given full hospital and health care facility visiting rights. This would include reviewing the patient's medical record and other personal health information. You can also request that your health care agent consult with certain designated individuals before key decisions are made.

Giving a health care agent your medical power of attorney does not grant them the authority to handle your finances. While a health care agent can be given that authority, it typically is not included within the scope of an advance directive. It is also important to note that a health care agent is not responsible for your medical expenses. Some people might be dissuaded from serving as a health care agent if they thought they would then become liable for paying the patient's medical bills.

When does a health care agent take over for the patient? This is also addressed in the forms. There are two instances that trigger the authority of a medical power of attorney. In the first, your health care agent takes over when your physician deems you incompetent to make medical decisions. The second arises when the patient, while still competent, authorizes the health care agent to take charge. For example, this might be useful if a patient were to undergo extensive surgery with a prolonged recovery period. The health care agent could make decisions while the patient is recovering but still weak.

A health care agent can also be given the power to authorize an autopsy, make anatomical gifts, and direct the disposition of the patient's remains. All of these can become important under certain circumstances.

Because Dave Eckhart had specified that Ellen was his health care agent, she was able to make tough decisions about his care. Ellen consulted with her family, but the final decisions were hers alone. Ellen followed Dave's wishes about organ donation, even if she might have disagreed with them or wouldn't have chosen organ donation for herself.

Many families struggle with these decisions when the patient has left no directions. Often arguments break out, sometimes with tears and yelling, leaving emotional scars that last for years. The designation of a health care agent spares the family the heavy burden of making group decisions at a very intense time. The patient's wishes are specified and respected, and this eases the stress for everyone.

# 10

## Palliative Care and Hospice

Lovers of truth—rise up! Let us go toward heaven. We've seen
enough of this world; it's time to see another.

RUMI

Palliative care and hospice: these two medical service modalities
come up in any conversation about end-of-life care. Sometimes the
terms are used interchangeably, but they are distinct and different.
The confusion comes in part because patients may receive hospice
care, palliative care, or both.

### Palliative Care

The Center to Advance Palliative Care provides the following definition:

> Palliative care is a medical specialty focused on improving
> overall quality of life for patients and families facing serious
> illness. Emphasis is placed on intensive communication, pain
> and symptom management, and coordination of care. Palliative
> care is provided by a team of professionals working together
> with the primary doctor. It is appropriate at any point in a
> serious illness and can be provided at the same time as treat-
> ment that is meant to cure.

What this means in practice is that a patient suffering from a
serious illness will have not only a medical team focusing on achiev-
ing a cure, but also a team focusing on symptoms, pain, and quality
of life. Until recently, a palliative care consultation was usually requested when all hope for a cure was gone and no further standard-

treatment options were available. This was often associated with the feeling of "giving up," and patients sometimes sensed that their doctor's focus had shifted to patients who could be helped. "Nothing more left to do, so let's send them to palliative or hospice care," is something I remember one colleague saying about a patient who was dying of end-stage heart disease.

But many nurses and physicians, including myself, have come to believe that palliative care should be considered as a regular and routine part of all medical care, from minor to the most severe problems. Often palliative care is employed at the end of life, but sometimes it is used in treating an illness that may last for years, such as multiple sclerosis.

Although it might not be called palliative care, the principle of attending to a patient's symptoms and quality of life is also employed in less extreme situations. Even when I set a broken arm in the emergency room, I prescribe pain medication and suggestions for how to get through daily living with one arm in a cast. The pain relief and care suggestions don't directly affect the speed with which the bone will knit back together, but a person's comfort and peace of mind are important contributors to healing and one's overall health.

In terms of serious illnesses, where the specialty field of palliative care is making great contributions, we are beginning to see benefits beyond what anyone might have predicted. A *New England Journal of Medicine* article entitled "Early Palliative Care for Patients with Metastatic Non-Small-Cell Lung Cancer" appeared in August 2010. "Metastatic" means cancer that has spread throughout the body, and "non-small-cell" refers to a type of lung cancer, one of the worst, and always fatal. In this study, palliative care was introduced early on in the medical care plan. The results were surprising: "Early palliative care led to significant improvements in both quality of life and mood. As compared to patients receiving standard care, patients receiving early palliative care had less aggressive care at the end of life but longer survival." Further, the "timely introduction of palliative care may serve to mitigate unnecessary and burdensome personal and society costs." In other words, those patients lived longer (about 2.7 months longer on average), were less depressed and/or happier, and the program saved everyone money. Sounds pretty good to me.

From a strictly scientific point of view, we can only speculate on the reasons why patients in this study lived longer. I believe this happened because the mind and body are interconnected at every level, although the mechanisms for the connections are not fully understood or appreciated. Perhaps living with less pain allows the body's immune system to fight the cancer better. Or maybe organs that would otherwise give out (like the heart, lungs, liver, kidneys), and whose failure leads directly to death, function more effectively when other symptoms and stresses are eased. Or maybe patients who are not in pain just eat better, providing their bodies with nutrients that keep them going longer.

In any case, the implications are clear. Palliative care should not be considered after "everything else has been tried." Rather, it should routinely be included early for patients with serious short-term or long-term illnesses.

Modern medical care can help cure disease. It can also help ease pain and suffering, and improve one's quality of life. We now know that these two objectives are fundamentally intertwined in our quest for longer and healthier lives.

## Hospice

The National Institutes of Health describes hospice care as "end-of-life care provided by health professionals and volunteers. They give medical, psychological, and spiritual support. The goal of the care is to help people who are dying have peace, comfort, and dignity. The caregivers try to control pain and other symptoms so a person can remain as alert and comfortable as possible. Hospice programs also provide services to support a patient's family."

Hospice is a concept of personalized medical care specifically for those at the end of life, when cures are no longer possible. Hospice affirms life and regards dying as a normal process. Hospice employs palliative care; it neither hastens nor postpones death. By Medicare's definition, hospice refers specifically to patients whose life expectancy is less than six months.

The hospice concept is not new, but it became reestablished in England in the 1950s. Since then, hospice has grown to over 4000 separate programs in the United States. Most of these are run by nonprofit organizations. Some are free standing; others are affiliated with other medical entities, such as hospitals. Today over 1.5 million Americans seek hospice services each year. Hospice is increasingly being recognized as an integral part of the health care delivery system.

The hospice team consists of doctors, nurses, social workers, pharmacists, clergy, nutritionists, and other practitioners and volunteers.

Hospice care can be delivered in a variety of settings, although most often in the patient's home. Initially, the hospice team meets with the patient and family members to assess their wishes, needs, and resources. Hospice workers will come to the patient's home to provide care, including education for family members, pain medication, nutrition, and counseling. Other important support services may be delivered as well, including respite care for home caregivers, medical supplies, special foods, and equipment. Volunteers and other practitioners may provide services as diverse as offering music therapy, reading aloud, running errands, or caring for pets, depending on a patient's needs.

Hospice care can also be provided in hospitals, nursing homes, and dedicated hospice facilities. Regardless of the setting, the goals are the same: to provide people who are dying with compassionate end-of-life care, to relieve pain and suffering, to offer support for family members, and to do so with respect for all concerned.

It takes a special person to choose hospice as a career. So often medical practitioners are trained to focus on "the cure." And sometimes we can cure. But when cures are no longer possible, some practitioners feel they have nothing more to offer. That doesn't have to be the case, and that's where hospice comes in.

I have witnessed hospice personnel at work and was most impressed with their patience: how they took time to carefully explain as much as possible about the dying process. Many patients don't fear death; after all, everyone knows it's coming some day. But we do fear dying. Will we suffer? Will we be helpless? Will we have our loved ones with us? Hospice has many excellent resources about what to expect when someone is dying. Even family members who are not primary caregivers can benefit from these.

Modern hospice care offers reassurance that the dying process will be managed as comfortably as possible. Family members are taught when to call for an ambulance and when not to. Training is offered in daily care tasks, such as bathing, dressing, and feeding. Pain medicines are used responsibly, as are sedatives and tranquilizers.

Of course, like any service, hospices vary in their quality. Be sure that all your questions are answered and issues addressed before engaging a particular hospice service.

But it's not all about medicine. Hospice brings a perspective on death and bereavement as a natural part of life's continuum. Too often people feel guilty or ashamed of their very normal feelings of sadness or fear or even relief. Sometimes all a patient or family member wants is the chance to talk and be heard without worrying that the conversation will scare everyone away.

Unfortunately, hospice care is often seen as something outside of the normal services of modern medical care, something to turn to when you've given up hope. Actually, hospice does provide hope: hope that the transition from this world to the next will be done utilizing all the tools modern medicine can offer, hope that the end of life will happen with comfort and dignity, hope that suffering will be eased.

## 11

# Abby Miller
## *A Better End*

I have seen that the prognosis may not be the reality any more
than the map is the territory or the blueprint the building.

RACHEL NAOMI REMEN, M.D.

Abby Miller was 54 years old when she got the diagnosis of
ovarian cancer, and it hit her hard. A guidance counselor by profession, she had enough presence of mind to know that she needed
some support even to hear the doctor's recommendations for treatment. "I wouldn't have remembered a word," she told her friend
Carol. "Once I heard 'cancer,' my brain kind of froze."

Abby had been divorced for over 10 years. Her son Josh lived
2000 miles away, where he'd recently started a new job. But she had
a large network of friends: some from work; some from church, her
book group, her knitting club; some she'd known ever since college.
Carol was the one she was closest to, and it was Carol whom she
invited to accompany her back to the doctor's office to hear what
lay ahead.

Dr. Reese was a breast cancer survivor herself, so she understood much of what Abby was going through. She told Abby that
each person was different and that making exact predictions was
impossible. But, at a minimum, Abby could expect several good
years ahead.

The three of them discussed options. Surgery? Chemotherapy?
Radiation? Cancer therapy has become increasingly individualized.
Cells are studied to determine which modalities or medications will
have the best chance of success with a particular type of tumor. This

process had already begun in Abby's case. The first step was surgery, to be followed by chemo. They scheduled the operation for the following week.

Abby didn't like to hide things. She called Josh in Texas, and she invited her closest friends to a gathering at her home that weekend. Their reactions were shock and dismay, followed by offers of help and support. Abby wasn't sure what kind of help she would need, but she appreciated knowing that they were there for her.

Prior to surgery, Abby obtained an advance directive and began to consider her options. It felt too soon to be making those decisions, but she decided to name Josh and Carol as joint health care agents. The rest she postponed until after surgery, when she would have a better idea of what she was up against.

Abby underwent a laparotomy, a full opening of the abdomen to get complete access to all internal organs. Her uterus, fallopian tubes, and ovaries were removed. At the same time, her other internal organs were examined, and samples of tissue were obtained to see if the cancer had spread.

Abby spent a few days in the hospital, recuperating from surgery. The biopsy results showed that the cancer had spread, but not far. She was a candidate for chemotherapy, but as chemo attacks the most rapidly growing cells, which include those that are repairing wounds, it would have to wait until after her surgical incisions healed. Josh wanted to fly out to be with her, but she assured him she was well taken care of. She told him to wait, to save his vacation and family-leave time for when she might need him more.

Her oncologist explained the typical course of her disease. Patients with her type of cancer usually responded well to the first round of chemo and would go into remission. When and if the cancer recurred, as it did in most cases like hers, a second round of chemo would be given; there would most likely be a good response, but not as good as the first one. This cycle would probably repeat two or three more times, but unless she was one of the few lucky ones whose cancer permanently disappeared, there would come a time when nothing more could be done.

Friends pitched in during her surgical recovery and first round of chemo, bringing meals to her at home and helping with errands. Carol discovered websites (lotsofhelpinghands.com and TakeThem AMeal.com) that helped to facilitate the sharing of tasks and schedules. Friends rotated visiting Abby, so that she was never alone for long periods, either in her house or during her treatments at the cancer clinic. Her job allowed flexible leave time, so Abby was able to continue to help the students she counseled. She joined a local support group of cancer patients, where she met other people in the same circumstances. Sharing emotions and life stories brought comfort.

The days after chemo were particularly hard. Abby was not so vain as to mind the resultant hair loss. She was amused that people thought she looked better in her new wig than she had with her own hair. But the nausea and fatigue were tough, and she struggled through those long days and nights.

Josh wanted her to get "everything possible" in terms of treatment, including any experimental or research protocols. He argued that "at least you will be helping someone else, if not yourself." That sounded good in theory, but when Abby was at the low point in her chemo cycle, the idea of going through horrible symptoms on the off chance that it would help some unknown person in the future felt unreasonable.

Abby returned to her advance directive. She struggled with the part about how much care to receive. She wanted every chance at survival, but she didn't want to suffer if there was no hope of recovery. At this point she certainly would want CPR if she experienced a cardiac or respiratory emergency. She finally decided that she would continue with treatment only as long as she could hope to live with meaningful functioning and a reasonable quality of life. But what did "a reasonable quality of life" mean for Abby?

Abby came to the conclusion that there were three things she especially loved that, for her, might define quality of life. The first was her dog, Mick, a scruffy poodle-terrier mix. Taking him for walks in the morning and evening was a highlight of her day, as was brushing his coat and cuddling with him in bed in the morning. Her second love was music. Abby liked all kinds of music, from opera to rock, and she especially loved Celtic folk music. The third was chocolate. Abby's favorite indulgence was two squares of dark chocolate after dinner. Along with the company of her loved ones, these daily rituals buoyed her mood through her illness. If she could no longer enjoy them, she would know that she was beyond a reasonable quality of life.

As the months progressed, Abby settled into the reality of living with cancer. Despite all the pain and nausea and anxiety, Abby eventually began to see herself as blessed in a peculiar way. She was no longer a victim; she was a survivor. Her appreciation for life was enhanced, and she savored every moment. Going to the movies with friends became a joyful experience, not just a night out. Things that had troubled her before became minor inconveniences, or even occasions for laughter. And Abby found a new capacity for patience. She had always been good at her counseling job, but her own struggles seemed to give her more empathy for her students and their problems.

Most precious of all, her relationship with her son deepened. They were able to speak of their love for each other in a way that hadn't been possible before. And Josh was able to talk more openly to his mother about his own life. Two years into her battle with cancer, Abby traveled cross-country for Josh's wedding to his girlfriend Emma. She shed bittersweet tears, grateful to be present at his marriage, but thinking of what she might not live to see.

This went on for four and a half years, through three rounds of chemo. Then Abby began to notice differences. Her pain was not responding as well to the pain medications. Her clothes hung on her thinning frame as she lost more weight. Breathing was getting harder, and she tired more quickly. Her walks with Mick the dog got shorter and less frequent. Eventually she hired a dog walker to take over.

One day she woke up with abdominal discomfort. This had happened before, but now it was worse. As the day progressed, she knew something was really wrong. Her belly bloated out, and the crampy pain increased. At three that afternoon, Carol took her to the emergency room. The diagnosis was a blocked bowel, a known complication of ovarian cancer and its treatment. A tube was put down her nose to ease the pressure, and Abby was admitted to the intensive care unit.

After two days, it was clear that surgery was required. The surgeon was confident that Abby would survive the operation. Without it, death was certain from the bowel blockage and the infection it would cause. Disoriented by the pain medications she'd been given, Abby struggled to understand what was going on. She could hardly imagine another operation. The first one had been tough enough, but she had been in pretty good shape back then. What would happen this time, when she was already in a weakened condition? She began to cry.

Who would decide what to do? At least one doctor was concerned that Abby was incompetent to make this decision, given her pain and heavy medication. Josh had flown in, and he and Carol considered the options. Was this a life-saving procedure or an effort at futile heroics? They agreed to go forward with the operation.

Abby awoke in the surgical recovery room. She was disoriented and groggy. The next few days were a fog, but she made a slow recovery. Eventually she was able to go home, but she resolved never to go through this again.

Four months after the surgery, the oncologist told her that the cancer was spreading again, and that the only possibility for stopping it lay with an untried experimental drug. Abby knew that she had reached the end. There was no timetable, but the doctor made it clear that death would most likely be soon.

Abby asked how the end might come. The doctor told her she might die from kidney or liver failure, as both organs were riddled with metastatic cancer. Or a growing tumor might erode a large blood vessel, causing internal bleeding. Or she'd develop an infection, probably pneumonia, as the final cause of death.

The financial paperwork had been completed, but Abby still had two issues to settle. The first was to update her advance directive to reflect that she no longer wanted 911 called in case of an emergency, nor did she want CPR given. The second issue was related: Where to die? Abby had spoken with others who had lost loved ones to cancer, and she had thought long and hard about what she wanted for herself.

She spoke with Josh and Carol about her decisions. She told them she was no longer a candidate for treatment. She didn't want to undergo any more surgery or chemo. She only wanted pain medicines, personal care, and comfort.

At first Josh was upset with her decision. Why refuse CPR? What about that experimental treatment? Why give up early? He and Emma were planning to have a child in the near future. Didn't Abby want to keep fighting to live long enough to see her first grandchild?

"Of course I want to know your children," Abby told him. "But this is not within my control. Or yours either." She brought out a folder and handed it to him. "I knew you and Emma would have children one day, and that I probably wouldn't be around to see them grow up. So I had myself videotaped. In here is a DVD with a message for my grandchildren. Things I want them to know but won't be there to share with them in person."

Through his tears, Josh nodded his acceptance. He could see how his mother was suffering. Sad as it was for him, in good conscience he couldn't ask her to prolong the ordeal.

Returning to her advance directive, Abby read what she had written: "I only want food and pain medicine, and if I get too weak to eat, I don't want artificial feeding. I want to be kept clean and comfortable, and I prefer that this care come as much as possible from those closest to me. I want to die at home, not in a hospital."

"I ask that my favorite music be present in my last days, and that Mick be allowed to be with me as long as possible. If my heart should stop beating or I stop breathing, stay with me and allow me to die in peace. I don't want you to ever feel guilty. By following my instructions, you are showing your love for me."

Abby hadn't come to these decisions lightly. Early on in Abby's illness, Dr. Reese had suggested that she meet with a nurse from the hospital's palliative care program. They had helped Abby deal with the discomforts that came with chemo and radiation therapy. They had also given her information about hospice programs available both in institutions and at home. Abby had already begun working with hospice and had found that the nurses and other staff members helped greatly in every aspect of her care. She appreciated their attention and professionalism. The care she got at home was excellent. Abby didn't want to die in an institution, no matter how homelike it tried to be.

As her last weeks approached, Abby talked with Josh and Carol about the kind of funeral she wanted. She didn't believe in spending money on an expensive casket or on embalming. Her faith that her spirit would live on after death had become stronger over the course of her illness, but she wanted her physical remains to be returned to the earth as quickly and naturally as possible.

Josh had been impressed by the wake held at home for Emma's uncle the previous year. It was comforting for Emma to pay her respects in the house where her uncle had lived, instead of in a funeral parlor. Older relatives had commented that wakes always used to be held at home.

Abby said that she would prefer a home wake, too, if Carol and her other friends were willing to do that for her. She liked the idea of her body being cared for at the end by the hands of those who loved her. Carol talked to the circle of Abby's friends, and they agreed that they would be honored to perform this last service for Abby. The burial would take place in the newly opened natural burial section of her church's cemetery, with a simple, engraved river stone to mark her grave.

Abby left it to Josh and Carol to plan the funeral service, only asking that some of her favorite pieces of music be played. She joked that given her wide circle of acquaintances, they had better talk to the minister about using the larger chapel.

It was only early November, but Abby decided to put up her Christmas tree. She had always loved decorating the house for the holidays, and she didn't know whether or not she'd make it to late

December. Her cancer had taught her to appreciate life during every moment, to give and receive happiness at every opportunity. She wanted her last weeks to be brightened by the lights and greenery, the ornaments collected and cherished over a lifetime.

During the next weeks Abby became too weak to leave her house, then too weak to leave her bedroom, and finally too weak to leave her bed. The hospice staff showed Josh, Carol, and the other helpers how to attend to Abby's hygiene needs, how to make the bed with her in it, and how to change her clothes easily.

With Mick nestled at her feet, Abby grew quiet and contemplative, listening to her favorite music, reading when she had the strength. She reflected on all the joys of her life and the people she had known. Sometimes she could almost feel the presence in the room of her own mother and father, who had died years before.

Friends and colleagues came to visit. Some would bring a special chocolate bar for her, and she would take a tiny bite, savoring the rich flavor. Frequently, this candy was the only thing she ate all day. Sometimes the visitors would just sit with her in silence, but often Abby took the opportunity to bestow a blessing on them or a piece of advice, and always a loving farewell.

One friend arranged for visits by a volunteer harpist who provided music for the very sick. The lilting tones of old Irish and Scottish melodies comforted Abby and everyone with her at the house.

As the days went by, her breathing became raspy. The hospice staff adjusted the dose of narcotics so Abby was comfortable and pain free without being overly sedated. Eventually she began to lapse in and out of consciousness, and the periods of sleep grew longer. She was calm and at peace. Then, one late afternoon as the sun was setting, she slowly slipped under the waves. With Josh holding her hand, she died, surrounded by loving friends.

When she had breathed her last, the hospice nurse bathed and dressed Abby's body. Carol and the others laid Abby out in her bed and prepared to welcome the friends who would stop by to pay their respects. The next day the funeral home came to lay Abby in her casket and transport her to the church for the funeral service and burial.

The end was still difficult for those left behind, but even as they grieved, they found comfort in the time they'd spent with Abby through the dying process. It made the loss more bearable. Her passing had been a deeply moving experience that would stay with them as long as they lived.

During the long drive back to their home with Mick, Josh and Emma talked about how much they'd appreciated Abby's attitude: her openness about her situation, her refusal to collapse into depression, and her joy in life no matter what was happening. She had given them the gift of seeing death as a meaningful part of the arc of a full life.

Abby achieved the better end, the best of both worlds. She took full advantage of modern medical science. She found a physician who was competent and compassionate. She allowed others to help her as necessary. She did not treat her disease as something to be ashamed of, but, on the other hand, she did not allow it to define her existence. She did not let it stop her from living and enjoying the good things around her. As a result, she survived longer than expected, and her positive attitude played a key role. When the end was in sight, she went out on her own terms. By doing so, she also provided a deeply meaningful life experience for those around her. If there is such a thing, hers was a beautiful death. With planning, more of us can have this experience.

## 12

# No Easy Answers
### Alzheimer's Disease and Dementia


We must build dikes of courage to hold back the flood of fear.
MARTIN LUTHER KING, JR.


Even if all the best efforts are made and everything is done right, sometimes there are no easy answers.

This is especially true—and most common—when someone has Alzheimer's disease or another form of dementia. Over half of all people who live past age 85 develop some form of dementia; it may be relatively mild and nonprogressive, or it may be severe and progressive. All dementia is produced by some type of injury to the brain. Whenever memory loss or confusion begins to interfere with daily living, it's important to obtain the correct diagnosis. For the majority of Americans with dementia, Alzheimer's disease is the cause. Dementia may also occur for other reasons, many of which can be treated. One cause that often can be successfully resolved is due to hydrocephalus, a build-up of fluid in the brain.

Alzheimer's disease, which results from brain degeneration, was first described in 1906 by the German physician Alois Alzheimer. While studying microscopic slides of brain tissue from patients with dementia who had died, he noticed similar plaques and tangles among the nerve cells of these different patients. Since the early twentieth century, the disease has become widely recognized and studied.

Alzheimer's disease can only be formally detected by examining brain tissue. Therefore, a diagnosis of Alzheimer's cannot be definitively confirmed without a brain biopsy, which is rarely performed on living patients, or an autopsy. But the constellation of symptoms is well established, and once the other possibilities are eliminated, Alzheimer's disease remains as the only likely candidate.

The cause of Alzheimer's is not known, although research has shown that certain lifestyle factors and treatable diseases can make a person prone to develop this type of dementia. These risk factors include smoking, excessive alcohol consumption, diabetes, high cholesterol, high blood pressure, insulin resistance, obstructive sleep apnea, thyroid abnormalities, periodontal disease, high-fat diets, and vitamin B12 and vitamin D deficiencies.

Whatever the cause, there is no specific treatment, though there are useful care plans that can be developed on an individualized basis. Over 5 million Americans are currently living with Alzheimer's disease; by 2050 that number will rise to 13.5 million.

The economic impact of Alzheimer's is staggering. Dementia affects the brain, but the body usually degenerates at a much slower rate, so it can take a long time until death arrives. During these years—or decades—as the dementia progresses, a person with dementia needs increasing amounts of care.

Often the symptoms begin insidiously. Forgetting where you left the house keys is something that happens to everyone. But with the slow onset of dementia, these rare events start to happen more and more often. Eventually an affected person begins to lose track of things that are not normally forgotten, such as a friend's name or one's own street address or how to do a simple calculation. Sometimes mood changes are the first indicator of dementia. Early on the patient is aware of the symptoms. Former president Ronald Reagan wrote movingly about this in a letter to the American people:

> I have recently been told that I am one of the millions of Americans who will be afflicted with Alzheimer's disease. Upon learning this news, Nancy and I had to decide whether as private citizens we would keep this a private matter or whether we would make this news known in a public way. In the past, Nancy suffered from breast cancer and I had my cancer sur-

geries. We found through our open disclosures we were able to raise public awareness. We were happy that as a result many more people underwent testing. They were treated in early stages and we were able to return to normal, healthy lives. So now, we feel it is important to share it with you. In opening our hearts, we hope this might promote greater awareness of this condition. Perhaps it will encourage a clearer understanding of the individuals and families who are affected by it. At the moment I feel just fine. I intend to live the remainder of the years God gives me on this earth doing the things I have always done. I will continue to share life's journey with my beloved Nancy and my family. I plan to enjoy the great outdoors and stay in touch with my friends and supporters. Unfortunately, as Alzheimer's disease progresses, the family often bears a heavy burden. I only wish there was some way I could spare Nancy from this painful experience. When the time comes, I am confident that with your help she will face it with faith and courage. In closing let me thank you, the American people, for giving me the great honor of allowing me to serve as your president. When the Lord calls me home, whenever that may be, I will leave with the greatest love for this country of ours and eternal optimism for its future. I now begin the journey that will lead me into the sunset of my life. I know that for America there will always be a bright dawn ahead. Thank you, my friends. May God always bless you.

President Reagan was able to afford the expensive individual care that helped keep him alive for years, while sparing his family many burdens. But for most Americans, dementia leads to great personal and economic hardship. It can cost many thousands of dollars each year to take care of a person with dementia.

Some people plan ahead by purchasing long-term-care insurance. This insurance can cover part of the cost of nursing home care, as well as home care. Premiums for such policies can be high, and they vary, depending on the level of coverage purchased. As with other insurance (such as for your car or your home), it is not possible to predict if the coverage will ever be needed.

For people with substantial financial resources, a continuing care retirement community (CCRC) is another way to plan ahead. Such facilities attract seniors who enjoy both mental and physical health; should the person later need extra care, he or she can move into the CCRC's assisted living facility or nursing care facility. Buying into a CCRC can cost anywhere from $60,000 to over $400,000, plus monthly fees that range from $1000 to $6000.

People without insurance or sizeable savings who have a catastrophic or long-term illness (such as dementia) are often forced to "spend down" virtually all their assets. For these people, a lifetime of accumulated funds is exhausted on health care. This system-imposed poverty eventually makes the person eligible for Medicaid, at which point health care costs will be paid for by the government. However, any provision for a spouse or any inheritance for children is gone. Some couples have been advised to file for divorce as soon as they learn one of them has Alzheimer's, in order to protect the healthy spouse's assets. You wouldn't think a situation could be made even more heartbreaking than receiving a diagnosis of Alzheimer's disease, but under our current health care regime, it is entirely possible.

Beyond the financial expenditures, the human costs are immeasurable. At first, most Alzheimer's patients can be taken care of at home. But as the disease takes its toll, symptoms often become worse. Stress on their caretakers mounts. A person who has Alzheimer's disease requires constant supervision, as well as help with the basics of daily living: feeding, getting dressed, bathing, and going to the bathroom. And as time goes by, that person's demands for attention grow. The patient may become incontinent, and unable to climb stairs or swallow solid food.

Eventually, medical issues arise. These sometimes are related to the dementia (such as developing an infection due to poor hygiene), but more often they are caused by the many diseases that afflict elderly people. In those situations, caretakers have to make medical decisions for their loved one. These are often very challenging. How can they tell what the patient is thinking and feeling? What is their inner life like when they can no longer speak? Are they happy or miserable? Do they have any awareness of what's going on? Is it time to make a move to a nursing home? When does "care" create more suffering than healing? More pain than comfort? For a loving spouse or adult child who has been designated as the health care agent for an Alzheimer's disease patient, these are difficult questions.

One such caregiver got a call in the middle of the night from the hospital's emergency department. His mother had fallen at the Alzheimer's disease facility where she lived and was taken to the hospital by ambulance. At the ER, the son learned that his mother's hip was broken. Although she had lost her ability to speak some years before, it was clear that she was in pain, and the only way to definitively relieve her pain was with surgery. But surgery would also be an agonizing experience, and she didn't have enough mental ability left to carry out a rehabilitation program after surgery. She'd never walk again, with or without the operation. Her son gave the go-ahead for surgery. His mother's hip was pinned, and she made it through a difficult convalescence. Since physical therapy was impossible, her eventual recovery only allowed her to sit up for a few minutes each day. Otherwise she was bedridden. Her son knows he did the only thing he could do, given all the circumstances, but he is far from content with the outcome.

I remember one patient with long-standing dementia. He spent each day at home under the watchful care of his wife. One day, she noticed that his face was drooping and one arm and leg were not moving. Being familiar with the signs of a stroke, she called 911 immediately, and the patient was brought to the ER. A CT scan confirmed blockage of an artery in the brain, and our stroke team was called in. Now came the hard part. To treat the patient with clot-busting drugs was risky and expensive, but they might minimize the effects of the stroke. Not to treat him meant that the stroke would progress, but there was no way to tell how far, or whether it would be fatal. Eventually the decision was made to treat him. In the end, the patient was left partially paralyzed, although maybe not as badly as if he had not been treated. But now he could no longer live at home. He was moved to a nursing home, where he died 10 months later of pneumonia. His wife still wonders if she did the right thing. Would it have been better to bring him back home and let him die of the stroke? But would he have died? Would he have suffered even more? These are impossible questions. There is simply no way to know the right answers.

In the above examples, luckily there was someone close to the patient who was able to make a decision. When there is no designated health care agent, situations can arise that challenge common sense. A dermatologist related the following story. He was called to a nursing home to see a 90-year-old woman with late-stage dementia who had developed a sore on her nose that wouldn't heal. He diagnosed basal cell cancer, a very slow-growing condition. His recommendation was to do nothing, given the patient's age and debility. More than likely the patient would die from other causes before the cancer would become dangerous. But because she had no advance directive, medical decisions were made for her by the county's social service department. And because they felt they had no right to do anything less than have her receive the maximum treatment available, the patient underwent several surgical procedures that were both expensive and uncomfortable. Given her condition, she had no understanding of what was being done to her. No one liked the situation, but no one could do anything to avoid it.

At the very least, given the prevalence of Alzheimer's disease, each of us ought to carefully consider what kind of care we'd want and under what circumstances. Advance directives are very helpful, but there are times when the forms simply cannot anticipate or account for every situation. Thus, although it may be difficult, talking candidly with our designated health care agent is essential. The answers won't be easy, but leaving these issues unaddressed will only make things worse for both the patient and the one who has to make the decisions.

There has been a recent drive to increase funding for research into causes, prevention, and treatment for Alzheimer's disease. We all can hope that these efforts will ease some of the human and medical dilemmas people currently face when confronted with this disease.

# 13

## Why Don't More People Have an Advance Directive?

Everybody has got to die, but I have always believed an exception would be made in my case.

WILLIAM SAROYAN

How many Americans have an advance directive? This question arose as I worked on public policy questions in the Maryland legislature relating to end-of-life care. I assumed it would be an easy question to answer. I was wrong. Although our public institutions collect data on almost every facet of health care, this is one area where data were scarce. While I have no proof, my guess is that this deficiency reflects yet another aspect of our culture's aversion to anything related to death and dying.

To answer the question, Professor Keshia Pollack (my colleague at the Johns Hopkins Bloomberg School of Public Health) and I designed a study to investigate the frequency of advance directives and people's attitudes toward them. Our study focused on Maryland, but as Maryland's population demographics mirror those of the United States, what we learned has broad application. And we discovered a number of interesting things (see Pollack, Morhaim, and Williams, "Public Perspectives on Advance Directives: Implications for State Legislative and Regulatory Policy," *Health Policy*, February 2010).

More than 80 percent of people over age 18 wanted their end-of-life wishes to be respected; however, only about a third of these people had completed advance directives. This suggests a significant gap. People had given thought to the question of their end-of-life care, but the majority hadn't completed the forms.

Why didn't people complete advance directives? About a quarter of the respondents said they didn't know about them. Others felt that they were too young or healthy to need them, or they were concerned about the cost, the complexity of the questions, or the time that might be required to complete the forms.

The age factor was significant. Younger people are much less likely than older people to have filled out an advance directive. It may *seem* unnecessary for a younger person to have such a document, but as we saw in chapter 7, the three most famous cases in American legal history concerning advance directives all involved people under the age of 30: Karen Ann Quinlan, Nancy Cruzan, and Terri Schiavo. Had these young women written advance directives, much heartache and legal hostility would probably have been avoided.

We asked people where they would prefer to get information about advance directives. Overwhelmingly, they wanted to obtain it from their doctors or other health care providers, rather than from attorneys, clergy, or online sources. While younger people, not surprisingly, were more comfortable locating information on the Internet, nearly everyone wanted the opportunity to review their decisions with medical professionals. This finding means that doctors, nurses, and the health care system have an important role to play.

The study also revealed significant differences among racial and cultural groups. Some groups were more likely than others to complete advance directives. For example, about twice as many whites as African Americans have completed advance directives. This disparity is important. It may be due to several factors, including cultural differences in family-centered decision making, one's level of trust in the health care system, and the quality of communication between health care professionals and patients. Research in other areas suggests that African Americans prefer to involve multiple family members, friends, and clergy in making health care decisions;

thus they may be more likely to designate a health care agent to co-ordinate that decision making, rather than state their own preferences in a living will.

The study clearly told us that Americans are concerned about end-of-life care. They worry about it, and they want to be involved. Too many Americans, however, are not sure how to proceed. Health care providers, attorneys, and others need to increase the public's awareness of how important these issues are and provide better information about them.

Advance directive forms are readily available, and they can be completed for free or at very low cost. Health care professionals must become more involved in discussing these issues with their patients, and this aspect of their practice needs to be supported. Ironically, that was the intent of the infamous "death panel" clause in the 2009 debate on health care reform. The clause would have given physicians modest but fair compensation for discussing this important issue with Medicare patients if the patients asked their doctors to do so.

Talking about advance directives needs to become a routine part of doctor-patient conversations, so that the topic becomes "normalized." The more ordinary or routine the topic becomes, the less scary it is. The reality, unfortunately, is that the subject of advance directives is not yet part of most medical exams. Until such time that it is, we must be the ones to take care of this issue for ourselves and for our loved ones.

If you're reading this book, you've obviously moved beyond the initial discomfort everyone feels about end-of-life issues. But what if you want to open the discussion with your spouse, a family member, or a friend? Many people are in deep denial on this subject. If you try to bring it up, they may shrug off your attempt with a joke or a rebuff. Physicians and nurses are not immune to denial, either. When this topic came up in a conversation with a friend who's a surgeon, he just grimaced and replied: "It'll all work out somehow or other." While what he said is undeniably true, the way it will work out may not be to his liking. Even with as much experience as he's had with illness and dying, he was simply unwilling to face the fact of his own eventual death.

One way to raise the topic is to make it part of a shared exercise. Aging with Dignity, the organization behind the "Five Wishes" format for an advance directive, suggests hosting a "Five Wishes" party. Invite all the adult members of your family plus any other interested friends, and give a copy of the "Five Wishes" document to everyone who comes. A gathering like this gives people the chance to ask questions, talk over the issues involved in choosing a health care agent, and explore the level of care they would prefer for themselves in different situations. Aging with Dignity provides an instructional DVD, called "Sharing the Gift," and a facilitator's guide that can be used to prepare the group for filling out the forms.

Whether or not you use the "Five Wishes" format, it's helpful to complete advance directives together with your family and friends. When you invite people to such a gathering, be sure you have the relevant forms available. Either fill out your own advance directive at the same time everyone else is, or bring your already completed advance directive with you for the others to read. Some people may want to have more time to consider the questions raised by an advance directive; in that case, you can schedule a follow-up meeting.

As our research showed, people want to take care of this kind of advance planning. Many of them just need someone to break the ice. That person can be you.

We are a diverse nation, and different strategies will apply in effectively reaching various groups. One group that is particularly under-served is the less affluent. People of greater financial means consult attorneys about their estate planning, and attorneys often raise the subject of advance directives at that time. But for those who don't need or can't afford estate planning, the topic may not come up until it's too late. I have seen the tragic results of this lack of advance preparation in many instances, such as that of Alberta Cole, whose story is told in chapter 3. Because so many people have no other way to learn about advance directives, a discussion about completing an advance directive should become a routine part of the relationship between patients and their health care providers. I believe that, while no one should ever be forced to have an advance directive, everyone should be given the information and the tools they need to have one if they want.

# 14

## Step Four

### *Legal and Other Decisions*

It is as natural to die as to be born.

FRANCIS BACON

For an advance directive to be valid, the person whose directive it is needs to sign and date the form. The legalities of the signature process vary from state to state, but the guiding principles are the same. Most states require one or two other adults to witness the maker's signature on the form with their own signatures. A witness can be almost anyone: a friend, a coworker, a neighbor. They don't need to see, know, or review the contents of your advance directive; they only need to see you sign the form. The only people who should *not* serve as witnesses are the persons designated to be your health care agents and anyone who stands to gain by your death through inheritance or as an insurance beneficiary. In addition, most states prohibit your health care provider from acting as a witness. These rules help to ensure the neutrality of the witnesses and to protect against a vulnerable patient being coerced either by a person who stands to gain from that individual's death or by a health care provider or the provider's employees.

In most states the witnesses are required to attest that they personally know the individual making the advance directive and that they believe that person to be of sound mind. In some states the signatures must be notarized by a notary public, as well. Notaries can be found in the phone book or through the Internet, and your bank or your lawyer's office may also have a notary on staff. The

Resources section of this book contains information about obtaining an advance directive form appropriate for your state.

What happens if you get sick while you are traveling? Or if you are taken to a hospital where you don't usually get care? How will your advance directive be found? These are real concerns, but there are solutions.

First, copies of your advance directive should be kept in several locations: your doctor's office, with your loved ones, and with whomever you have designated as your health care agent. You may also want to carry a copy (or a reduced-size version) with you when you travel.

Second, if you do receive regular care at an institution such as a hospital, nursing home, or hospice, they will want to have a copy. Just be sure that you send them any updated forms, so they always have your latest version.

Despite their best intentions, health care providers are not always as well informed as they should be about the legalities of advance directives. This is because advance directives are still relatively uncommon. As an emergency room doctor, I might see only a handful in a year among the hundreds of seriously ill people I treat.

This is an area where patients need to become their own advocates. Patients should educate themselves as to the legal requirements in their state and make sure they have an updated and legally signed form. In fact, you may need to educate your health care providers. As advance directives become more common, providers will become more familiar with them, and implementation will become more routine.

Third, there are some states (Arizona, Idaho, Louisiana, Montana, North Carolina, Vermont, and Washington State) that offer an Advance Directive Registry to their citizens. On a purely voluntary basis, citizens can file their advance directive with the state's registry, where it is kept confidential and can only be accessed by appropriate persons. I believe that every state should make this service available.

Finally, entities such as the U.S. Living Will Registry will maintain your living will on file for a modest fee, and they will make it available if it is needed.

An advance directive is only useful if it can be found and applied. Be sure to take care of the important step of making sure your advance directive is up to date, available, and accessible.

## Organ Donation

Every year organ transplantation helps thousands of people to live longer and more productive lives. (Organ donation information can be found at the websites listed in the Resources section.)

Some advance directive forms include an optional part relating to organ donation. Within this section, there are several choices. One can specify that only certain organs be used—such as skin (to treat people who have been severely burned) or corneas (the clear surface tissue of the eye that can be transplanted to restore sight)—or that all usable organs can be transplanted. Donations may also be made for research and educational purposes.

Decisions about organ donation do not have to be part of an advance directive. Many people make those choices using other forms or have their preference noted on their driver's license. However one's donor status is documented, when a decision to harvest organs is made, experts review the patient's wishes and medical condition, and discuss organ donation with family members.

I have witnessed the life-giving and sight-restoring results of organ transplants, and I subscribe to the message of the bumper sticker that tells us: "Don't take your organs to Heaven. We need them right here on Earth."

## Dust to Dust

Eventually our bodies must go somewhere after we die. Some people include instructions for what they want to happen to their earthly remains as part of their advance directives. There are several options, depending on your beliefs, preferences, traditions, and means.

## Whole Body Donation

Some people arrange to donate their bodies to science or medical education. These bodies help physicians and other health care professionals learn human anatomy. The anatomy lab is the first important class in medical school. Without the bodies that are donated for medical education, it would be difficult, if not impossible, for doctors to gain a comprehensive understanding of human anatomy in all its beauty and complexity.

For some people the idea of body donation seems ghoulish; for others, there is comfort in knowing that their bodies are helping others to learn. Instructors pass on to students the tradition of treating the donated bodies with respect in the medical school anatomy lab. If you choose to donate your body to medical science, it's best to make arrangements in advance with a medical school. Many schools hold a memorial service for family and friends to remember the deceased. There is no charge for donating a body or for the memorial service.

## Funerals

Most Americans choose to have a funeral home handle and dispose of their remains, either through burial or cremation. Funerals vary in price; in 2009 the average American funeral cost between $8000 and $10,000. Cremations averaged $2000, not including any costs associated with disposing of the cremated remains in a burial vault or a cemetery plot.

There are serious environmental issues connected with the standard funeral options. One is the higher-than-normal cancer rates in mortuary and casket-manufacturing workers caused by the toxic chemicals in embalming fluid and the finishes used on most coffins. These same chemicals go into the ground, along with the metal or hardwood coffins used by most Americans. In addition, almost all U.S. cemeteries insist that the casket be interred in a concrete vault. This is not legally required, but it allows for ease of landscape maintenance.

According to the Casket and Funeral Association of America, each year in the United States, cemetery burials involve 827,000 gallons of embalming fluid and caskets containing 92,000 tons of steel, 2700 tons of copper and bronze, and 30+ million board-feet of hardwoods. Cremation and burial vaults use 1,640,000 tons of reinforced concrete and 14,000 tons of steel. Once these materials are placed underground, they can no longer be used or recycled. To look at these numbers in a different way, as Mark Harris wrote in his book, *Grave Matters*: "The amount of wood from coffins in a ten-acre cemetery is enough to build 40 houses, and there's enough concrete to build swimming pools for all of them."

Cremation also has environmental drawbacks. It releases carbon monoxide, sulfur dioxide, and other greenhouse gases and persistent organic pollutants into the atmosphere. Each cremation uses the energy equivalent of a 4800-mile car trip.

For these and other reasons, including financial ones, more Americans are forgoing embalming and expensive caskets and opting for simpler and more natural ways to return their physical remains to the earth.

Most Americans are not aware that in most states there is no legal requirement to use a funeral home at all. In fact, a hundred years ago, funeral homes were rare. A person died and was laid out at home, visitors paid their respects, and the person was buried in the churchyard or family plot behind the house. Today this tradition is no longer common, but it is still legal in almost every state. Once a proper death certificate is obtained, families can dispose of the body by burial on private property. The laws and regulations on this vary from locality to locality. If this approach interests you, you should investigate the particular statutes and regulations for where you want the burial to take place.

Likewise, a home funeral or wake (like the one described in Abby Miller's story in chapter 11) is an option for some. There is also a growing movement to return to natural burial practices, either in the "green sections" of established cemeteries or in new, natural burial preserves. You can find out more about home funerals and natural burial by contacting the alternative funeral and burial websites listed in the Resources section.

## Ceremonies

Whatever method you choose for disposing of your body or the body of a loved one, survivors usually find comfort in a formal ceremony of remembrance. Whether at a solemn funeral mass in a cathedral or at a simple memorial service at home, friends and family have the opportunity to remember the deceased and say goodbye. Every religious faith has traditions about memorial commemorations. While some people feel that these ceremonies are not needed in our modern scientific world, I believe we should not disregard the collective psychological wisdom of the human race. Once death has occurred, our primary focus turns to bringing comfort to the survivors.

# 15

## Speaking Personally

> Security is mostly a superstition. It does not exist in nature, nor do the children of men as a whole experience it. Avoiding danger is no safer in the long run than outright exposure. Life is either a daring adventure, or nothing.
>
> HELEN KELLER

Sometimes people ask about my personal views on death and dying. What are my values when it comes to end-of-life choices? What would I take into account, or what would I want my health care agent to take into account, if such decisions need to be made?

The first question for me—as for many people—would be: Is my mind working? Do I have consciousness, even if it is somewhat impaired?

Second, what's going on with my body? Am I in pain? How much care do I need? Have I become a burden to my loved ones? Am I so debilitated that every bodily function needs support?

And third, what is the context of my life? Am I surrounded by family and friends? Or am I living in an isolated situation in an institution?

If my mind is functional and my pain or discomfort is tolerable, then I would want to be kept alive as long as possible, using every modality reasonably available. But if I can only look forward to bare survival, without mental capacity or a reasonable hope of regaining functions, or if I'm in extreme pain, then I would only want those measures taken that would keep me comfortable. In such a case I would not want artificial nutrition to prolong my life.

Just about every health provider I know who works in emergency or critical care medicine has completed an advance directive. Why? Because we've seen what happens when people don't. We've seen the people who get something called "care," when it's really closer to torture. We've also seen amazing cures and recoveries. And while we know that medicine is not an exact science, we are certain that there comes a time when enough is enough—when we cross that line between meaningful care and the humility to let nature take its course.

I urge everyone over the age of 18 to complete an advance directive. The websites in the Resources section will help you find the forms you'll need. Take the time to think about what you would want, consult with people whose advice you respect, and then make sure the forms are complete and are legally valid. Be sure to let other people know where your advance directive is kept. If possible, give a copy to your doctor and your health care agent. And, should your wishes or circumstances change, update your advance directive as often as you like.

The dollar cost of completing, legalizing, and distributing these forms is minimal, or even free, but the benefits are invaluable.

I make many presentations on a variety of medical topics, including a health policy series at the Johns Hopkins Bloomberg School of Public Health. This series covers a broad range of health care policy topics. Most of the people attending are graduate students at the school, who comprise a diverse group of men and women from this country and abroad, generally in their 20s and 30s. Many already have a graduate degree in another field. There are doctors, nurses, lawyers, social workers, scientists, and people who work in business or public policy fields. This combination of professions leads to some interesting discussions about ethics, economics, and politics, as well as medical science.

When we cover the topic of end-of-life care, I ask how many students have completed an advance directive. Usually just a few hands go up—and never more than 20 percent of the audience. I then ask the students to find suitable forms and go through the process of completing them. I think it's important to have a personal experience, when possible, if one is going to discuss and take a position on the decisions of others.

Completing an advance directive more closely connects a person with life and death. The process helps each of us confront our basic values. My students come back to me over the course of the series and thank me for pushing them into this experience. Many have told me that completing an advance directive has changed their view of the health care system and the people in it. They develop a better rapport with patients and health care providers, and an appreciation of the difficult choices that are involved. One said: "I now have a greater sense of empathy for every human being."

I wrote this book because I believe that each of us needs to learn how to survive, and eventually to die, in today's modern medical world.

The consequences of our decisions can be far reaching. Will our loved ones spend years at our bedside agonizing over decisions? Will arduous and painful—but ultimately futile—treatment be administered because no one was there to direct our care? Will end-of-life expenses bankrupt our family? Will family conflicts erupt because we did not take the time to express our wishes when we were able to do so? It doesn't have to be this way. The actions we take when it comes to making sure we express our wishes regarding our end-of-life care greatly affect the happiness, well-being, and finances of those nearest to us. Death is universal, but families who have lived through a more deliberately and thoughtfully planned process during their loved one's transition from life are better off. Not only are they often able to bond with each other in the face of their grief, but, years later, they look back with reverence on this experience.

I believe that, as a culture, we are in denial of death. We desperately need to enhance our empathy with our fellow beings as they move through this passage. As psychotherapist Josefine Speyer has noted, "when we embrace death as a part of life, we also embrace the ill, the dying, and the bereaved as partners in living."

We need to seize that best of both worlds. First, we should

strive for life and health for everyone with all the tools that science and ingenuity and compassion can offer. Then, when the end is approaching—as it must for all of us—we must use that same science, ingenuity, and compassion to bring comfort and dignity to the dying and their survivors.

We have been given a gift: the opportunity to actively participate in the drama of life's final passage. To prepare for it, we need to take action—carefully considering, and then completing, an advance directive.

# Resources

........................................................................

*Websites that provide information about specific topics covered in this book are listed first below. State-by-state listings of advance directive websites appear after the topical websites.*

## For More Information

### General

"Five Wishes"
www.agingwithdignity.org
    "Five Wishes" has become America's most popular living will, because it is written in everyday language. It helps structure important conversations about care in times of serious illness. It meets the legal requirements in 42 states. In the remaining eight (Alabama, Indiana, Kansas, New Hampshire, Ohio, Oregon, Texas, and Utah), a completed "Five Wishes" form can be attached to the form required by the state.

Congressional Research Service Report on End-of-Life Care
www.opencrs.com/document/R40235/
    In February 2009 the Congressional Research Service produced a report that provides an excellent and comprehensive summary and analysis of end-of-life care. It covers services, costs, ethics, and quality of care.

### Palliative Care

www.getpalliativecare.org
    Consult this website (and see chapter 10) for information about palliative care.

*Hospice*

www.nhpco.org
www.hospicenet.org
www.hospicefoundation.org
These websites offer information about hospice care (also see chapter 10).

*Organ Donation*

Two helpful resources provide complete information and answer frequently asked questions (FAQs) about all aspects of organ donation.

The first is www.organdonor.gov, an official U.S. government website managed by the U.S. Department of Health and Human Services. It points out that "each organ and tissue donor saves or improves the lives of as many as 50 people. Giving the 'Gift of Life' may lighten the grief of the donor's own family. Many donor families say that knowing other lives have been saved helps them cope with their tragic loss."

The second site is www.donatelife.net. Donate Life America is comprised of national organizations and 47 local affiliates across the United States that coordinate donation-related activities at the grassroots level.

*Alternative Funeral and Burial Resources*

The Funeral Consumers Alliance is a nonprofit organization dedicated to protecting a consumer's right to choose a meaningful, dignified, affordable funeral. It provides information about funeral options, and serves as a consumer advocate for legal and regulatory reform, at www.funerals.org.

Home Funerals
A number of groups exist that support home funerals or wakes. Among the best are Crossings: Caring for Our Own at Death at www.crossings .net, and the National Home Funeral Alliance at www.homefuneral alliance.org.

Natural Burial
Natural burial organizations promote burials that are ecologically friendly and less expensive than conventional American funerals. Two

helpful sites are the Centre for Natural Burial at www.naturalburial.coop and the Green Burial Council at www.greenburialcouncil.org.

Body Donation
Body donations can contribute to medical research and medical education. Donation also avoids funeral and burial expenses. Each state has its own anatomical board that operates body donation programs. Almost all of these boards are affiliated with a university or medical school. A complete listing can be found at www.med.ufl.edu/anatbd/usprograms .html.

Other resources include:
www.anatomicgift.com
www.sciencecare.com
www.biogift.org

### Advance Directives

*In compiling this state-by-state listing of websites that can help you obtain the forms you need in your home state, preference was given to government agencies as sources of information when possible. Additional information was drawn from credible nongovernmental sources (such as state bar associations or medical associations) when appropriate or necessary. The websites were current at the time this book went to the printer. If you do not find what you are looking for by using the web addresses provided here, please contact your state attorney general's office by e-mail or telephone and ask for a set of advance directive documents for your state.*

#### Alabama

Advance Directives (Alabama Medicaid Agency)
www.medicaid.state.al.us/resources/advance_directives.aspx

Advance Directives (Alabama Hospital Association)
www.alaha.org/resources.aspx?id=33

Life Plan: Planning Ahead for Your Future Health Needs (Alabama State Bar)
www.alabar.org/public/lifeplan.cfm

Forms: Advance Directive for Health Care—Living Will and Health Care Proxy [the two websites have identical forms] www.alaha.org/uploadedFiles/Resources/advdirective.pdf (Alabama Hospital Association) www.alabar.org/members/consumer-guide_forms_8_2008.pdf (Alabama Bar Association)

*Alaska*

Advance Directives (Department of Health and Social Services) www.epi.hss.state.ak.us/pubs/guide/Guide_16.htm

Form: Advance Directives for Health Care (Department of Health and Social Services) www.hss.state.ak.us/pdf/advancedirective.pdf

*Arizona*

Life Care Planning (Attorney General's Office) www.azag.gov/life_care/index.html

Guide to Filing Advance Directives (Office of the Secretary of State) www.azsos.gov/Adv_Dir/guide.pdf

Arizona Advance Directive Registry (Office of the Secretary of State) www.azsos.gov/Adv_Dir/

Forms: Durable Health Care Power of Attorney, Living Will, Pre-Hospital Medical Directive (Attorney General's Office) www.azag.gov/life_care/index.html

*Arkansas*

Advanced Directives—Aging with Dignity (Department of Human Services/Arkansas Innovative Performance Program) www.medicaid.state.ar.us/Download/general/units/oltc/training/addirect.pdf

Form: Living Will and Durable Power of Attorney for Health Care (Department of Human Services/Arkansas Innovative Performance Program) www.medicaid.state.ar.us/Download/general/units/oltc/training/addirect.pdf

*California*

Advance Health Care Directives (Office of the Attorney General)
www.ag.ca.gov/consumers/pdf/AHCDS1.pdf

Your Living Will (California Medical Association)
www.cmanet.org/publicdoc.cfm/7

Form: Advance Health Care Directive (Office of the Attorney General)
www.ag.ca.gov/consumers/pdf/ProbateCodeAdvancedHealthCare
DirectiveForm-fillable.pdf

Form: Advance Health Care Directive (California Hospital Association)
www.calhospital.org/sites/chadocuments.org/files/file-attachments/
Forms3.pdf

*Colorado*

Advance Directives (Department of Regulatory Agencies)
www.dora.state.co.us/insurance/senior/stern12.pdf

Colorado Advance Directive Program [only addresses CPR] (Department
of Public Health and Environment)
www.cdphe.state.co.us/em/Operations/CPRDirectives/index.html

Advance Directive Medical Information (Colorado Bar Association)
www.cobar.org/index.cfm/ID/1073/dpwfp/Advance-Medical-Directive
-Information

Form: Declaration as to Medical or Surgical Treatment (Colorado Bar
Association)
www.cobar.org/Docs/livingwill1003.pdf

Form: Patient's or Authorized Agent's Directive to Withhold Cardiopul-
monary Resuscitation (CPR) (Department of Public Health and
Environment)
www.cdphe.state.co.us/em/Operations/CPRDirectives/template.pdf

### Connecticut

Connecticut's Living Will Laws (Office of the Attorney General)
www.ct.gov/ag/cwp/browse.asp?a=2130&bc=0&c=19278

Forms: Information Pamphlet, Living Will, Advance Directives Combined
Form, Appointment of Health Care Representative (Office of the Attorney
General)
www.ct.gov/ag/lib/ag/health/yourrightstomakehealthcaredecisions2006
version.pdf

### Delaware

Advance Directives/Living Wills (Department of Health and Social
Services)
http://dhss.delaware.gov/dsaapd/advance.html

Form: Advance Health Care Directive (Department of Health and Social
Services)
http://dhss.delaware.gov/dsaapd/files/advancedirective.pdf

### District of Columbia

Form: Advance Directive (District of Columbia Hospital Association)
www.dcha.org/Publications/AdvanceDirective.pdf

### Florida

FAQ about Advance Directives (The Florida Bar)
www.floridabar.org/TFB/TFBResources.nsf/Attachments/FF083234399
AD67685256E28005CAC3E/$FILE/LivingWillsFAQs.pdf?Open
Element

End-of-Life Issues (Agency for Health Care Administration)
www.floridahealthfinder.gov/reports-guides/end-life-issues.aspx

Health Care Advance Directives (Agency for Health Care
Administration)
www.floridahealthfinder.gov/reports-guides/advance-directives.aspx

Forms: Living Wills, Health Care Surrogates, and Advance Directives (The Florida Bar)
www.floridabar.org/tfb/TFBConsum.nsf/0a92a6dc28e76ae58525700a005dod53/1f6f8a67f5a2382d8525770e005747fd!OpenDocument

Forms: Living Will, Designated Surrogates (Office of the Attorney General)
http://myfloridalegal.com/pages.nsf/Main/B18C541B29F7A7F885256FEF0044C13A

Forms: Living Will, Designation of Health Care Surrogate, Donor Form (Florida Agency for Health Care Administration)
www.floridahealthfinder.gov/reports-guides/advance-directives.aspx

### Georgia

Georgia Advance Directive for Health Care (Department of Human Services)
http://aging.dhr.georgia.gov/DHR-DAS/GEORGIA ADVANCE DIRECTIVE FOR HEALTH CARE-07.pdf

Form: Georgia Advance Directive for Health Care (Department of Human Services)
http://aging.dhr.georgia.gov/DHR-DAS/GEORGIA ADVANCE DIRECTIVE FOR HEALTH CARE-07.pdf

### Hawaii

Deciding "What If?" (City and County of Honolulu, Elderly Affairs Division/University of Hawaii)
www.hawaii.edu/uhelp/files/DecidingWhatIf_06.pdf

Health Care Decisions (Department of Health)
http://hawaii.gov/health/disability-services/neurotrauma/key-services -health.html

Form: Advance Health Care Directive (Executive Office on Aging)
http://hawaii.gov/health/eoa/Docs/AHCD.pdf

*Idaho*

Living Wills and Idaho's Natural Death Act (Office of the Attorney General)
www.ag.idaho.gov/livingWills/livingWills_index.html

Advance Directives (Department of Health and Welfare)
www.ag.idaho.gov/livingWills/livingWills_index.html

Health Care Directive Registry (Secretary of State)
http://sos.idaho.gov/general/hcdr.htm

Forms: Living Will and Durable Power of Attorney (Secretary of State)
http://sos.idaho.gov/general/FORMS/LivingWill_DurablePowerOf Attorney.pdf

Form: Idaho Health Care Directive Registry (Secretary of State)
http://sos.idaho.gov/general/FORMS/Registry_Form.pdf

*Illinois*

Statement of Illinois Law on Advance Directives (Department of Public Health)
www.idph.state.il.us/public/books/advin.htm

Advance Directives (Department of Aging)
www.state.il.us/aging/1abuselegal/legal_adv-directives.htm

Forms: Living Will, Power of Attorney for Health Care, Do Not Resuscitate (Department of Public Health)
www.idph.state.il.us/public/books/advin.htm

Form: Power of Attorney for Health Care (Department of Aging)
www.state.il.us/aging/1news_pubs/publications/poa_healthcare.pdf

Form: Living Will (Department of Aging)
www.state.il.us/aging/1news_pubs/publications/poa_will.pdf

*Indiana*

Advance Directives (Department of Health)
www.in.gov/isdh/files/advanceddirectives.pdf

No state-specific forms provided.

*Iowa*

Advance Directives (Department of Aging)
www.aging.iowa.gov/Documents/Publications/GiftofPeaceofMind.pdf

Living Wills (Iowa State Bar Association)
http://iabar.net/displaycommon.cfm?an=1&subarticlenbr=152

Powers of Attorney for Health Care Decisions (Iowa State Bar
Association)
http://iabar.net/displaycommon.cfm?an=1&subarticlenbr=154

Forms: Declaration Relating to Life-Sustaining Procedures (Living Will)
and Durable Power of Attorney for Health Care Decisions (Medical
Power of Attorney) (Iowa State Bar Association)
http://iabar.net/associations/4664/files/ISBAForms/ISBA_Form123
_032010.pdf

Forms: Durable Power of Attorney for Health Care and Living Will
(Department of Aging)
www.aging.iowa.gov/Documents/Publications/GiftofPeaceofMind
.pdf

*Kansas*

A Guide to Legal Issues in Life-Limiting Conditions (Department on
Aging)
www.agingkansas.org/Publications/Other/Guide_to_Legal_Issues_in
_LifeLimiting_Conditions.pdf

Advance Directives (Kansas Health Ethics)
www.kansashealthethics.org/advDir.php

Living Wills and Durable Power of Attorney for Health Care (Kansas Bar Association)
www.ksbar.org/public/public_resources/pamphlets/living_wills.shtml

Forms: Living Wills and Durable Power of Attorney for Health Care (Kansas Bar Association)
www.ksbar.org/public/public_resources/pamphlets/living_wills.shtml

Forms: Durable Power of Attorney for Healthcare Decisions, Living Will, Do No Resuscitate Directive (Kansas Health Ethics)
www.kansashealthethics.org/advDir.php

### Kentucky

Living Will Directive and Health Care Surrogate Designation in Kentucky (Legislative Research Commission)
http://lrc.ky.gov/Lrcpubs/LivingWill.pdf

Kentucky Living Will Packet (Office of the Attorney General)
http://ag.ky.gov/NR/rdonlyres/2DA643B3-B474-44B6-8A7E-9EDC7 B88FD1C/o/living_will_packet.pdf

Living Wills in Kentucky (Office of the Attorney General)
http://ag.ky.gov/civil/consumerprotection/livingwills.htm

Form: Living Will Directive (Legislative Research Commission)
http://lrc.ky.gov/Lrcpubs/LivingWill.pdf

Form: Living Will Directive and Health Care Surrogate Designation (Office of the Attorney General)
http://ag.ky.gov/NR/rdonlyres/2DA643B3-B474-44B6-8A7E-9EDC7 B88FD1C/o/living_will_packet.pdf

### Louisiana

Living Will Registry (Secretary of State)
www.sos.louisiana.gov/tabid/208/Default.aspx

Form: Living Will Declaration (Secretary of State)
www.sos.louisiana.gov/tabid/208/Default.aspx

### Maine

Taking Charge of Your Health (Office of the Department of Health and Human Services)
www.maine.gov/dhhs/oes/resource/rit2chew.htm

Form: Health Care Advance Directive (Office of the Department of Health and Human Services)
www.maine.gov/dhhs/oes/resource/adf.pdf

### Maryland

Advance Directives (Office of the Attorney General)
www.oag.state.md.us/Healthpol/AdvanceDirectives.htm

Form: Maryland Advance Directive (Office of the Attorney General)
www.oag.state.md.us/Healthpol/adirective.pdf

### Massachusetts

Advance Care Planning (Commission on End of Life Care)
www.endoflifecommission.org/end_pages/advance_care.htm

Health Care Proxy Information, Instructions and Form (Massachusetts Medical Society)
www.massmed.org/AM/Template.cfm?Section=Home&TEMPLATE=/CM/HTMLDisplay.cfm&CONTENTID=10737

Form: Health Care Proxy (Massachusetts Medical Society)
www.massmed.org/AM/Template.cfm?Section=Home6&TEMPLATE=/CM/ContentDisplay.cfm&CONTENTID=2570

### Michigan

Advance Directives (State Bar of Michigan)
www.michbar.org/elderlaw/adpamphlet.cfm

Advance Directives (Department of Community Health/Michigan State Long Term Care Ombudsman Program)
www.michigan.gov/documents/mdch/mdch_AdvanceDirectivesPamphlet_196639_7.doc

Forms: Durable Power of Attorney for Health Care, Living Will, Do-Not-Resuscitate Order (Department of Community Health/Michigan State Long Term Care Ombudsman Program)
www.michigan.gov/documents/mdch/mdch_AdvanceDirectivesPamphlet_196639_7.doc

Forms: Durable Power of Attorney for Health Care, Living Will, Do-Not-Resuscitate Declaration (State Bar of Michigan)
www.michbar.org/elderlaw/adpamphlet.cfm

### Minnesota

Questions and Answers about Health Care Directives (Department of Health)
www.health.state.mn.us/divs/fpc/profinfo/advdir.htm

Advance Directives (Minnesota Medical Association)
www.mnmed.org/EventsandServices/ResourcesforYourPatients/Advance
Directives/tabid/1462/Default.aspx

Form: Health Care Directive (Board on Aging)
www.mnaging.org/advisor/directive.htm

Form: Health Care Directive (Minnesota Medical Association)
www.mnmed.org/Portals/mma/PDFs/MN-Health-Care-Directive.pdf

### Mississippi

Patient Self Determination Act/ Mississippi Advance Health-Care Directive (Department of Health)
http://unite.msdh.state.ms.us/msdhsite/_static/resources/75.pdf

Form: Advance Health-Care Directive (Department of Health)
http://unite.msdh.state.ms.us/msdhsite/_static/resources/75.pdf

### Missouri

Living Wills and Other Advance Directives (The Missouri Bar)
www.mobar.org/99b8baa9-d44d-4756-9b40-fcdf1dd91ceb.aspx

Life Choices (Office of the Attorney General)
http://ago.mo.gov/publications/lifechoices/lifechoices.pdf

Missouri Law Regarding a Patient's Right to Make Health Care
Treatment Decisions (Department of Health and Senior Services)
http://health.mo.gov/seniors/ombudsman/pdf/ABriefSummaryHAMMER
BROCHURE.pdf

Forms: Durable Power of Attorney for Health Care, Health Care
Directive (The Missouri Bar)
http://members.mobar.org/pdfs/publications/public/dpa.pdf

Form: Durable Power of Attorney for Health Care Choices & Health
Care Choices Directive (Office of the Attorney General)
http://ago.mo.gov/publications/lifechoices/lifechoices.pdf

### Montana

Advance Health Care Directives (Department of Justice)
www.doj.mt.gov/consumer/consumer/advancedirectives.asp

Advance Medical Directives (Department of Public Health and Human
Services)
www.dphhs.mt.gov/sltc/services/aging/legal/documents/legaladvanced
directives.shtml

Montana End-of-Life Registry (Department of Justice)
https://app.mt.gov/registry/

Form: My Choices Advance Directive (Department of Justice)
www.doj.mt.gov/consumer/consumer/forms/advancedirective.pdf

Form: Declaration of Living Will Appointment (Department of Public
Health and Human Services)
www.dphhs.mt.gov/sltc/services/aging/legal/documents/livingwill
.pdf

Form: Montana End-of-Life Registry—Consumer Registration Agreement
(Department of Justice)
www.doj.mt.gov/consumer/consumer/forms/eolregistrationagreement
consumer.pdf

### Nebraska

Surrogate Decision Making in Nebraska (Department of Health and
Human Services)
www.hhs.state.ne.us/ags/docs/miltc.pdf

Living Will and Durable Power of Attorney for Health Care (Nebraska
Bar Association)
www.thompson.law.pro/wp-content/uploads/vlp-livingwillbrochure.pdf

Forms: Living Will, Power of Attorney for Health Care (Department of
Health and Human Services)
www.hhs.state.ne.us/ags/advdir.htm

### Nevada

Advance Directives (Department of Health and Human Services)
http://dhcfp.state.nv.us/advancedirectives.htm

Advance Directives (Nevada Center for Ethics and Health Policy,
University of Nevada, Reno)
www.unr.edu/ncehp/ADs.html

Living Will Lockbox (Secretary of State)
http://nvsos.gov/online/nadr/

Forms: Declaration and Durable Power of Attorney for Healthcare
Decisions (Department of Health and Human Services)
http://dhcfp.state.nv.us/HIPAA/NV Law Concerning Advanced Directives
.pdf

Form: Living Will Online Completion for Nevadans (Nevada Center for
Ethics and Health Policy, University of Nevada, Reno)
www.nvlivingwill.com/index.php

Form: Living Will Lockbox Registration Agreement (Secretary of State)
http://nvsos.gov/Modules/ShowDocument.aspx?documentid=155

*New Hampshire*

Advance Care Planning Guide (Foundation for Health Communities/
New Hampshire Partnership for End-of-Life Care)
www.healthnh.com/fhc/initiatives/performance/eol/ACPG 2007
revisions.pdf

Advance Directives and Do Not Attempt Resuscitation (Foundation for
Health Communities/New Hampshire Partnership for End-of-Life Care)
www.healthnh.com/fhc/initiatives/performance/eol/EOLManual.php

End-of-Life Care Reports (Foundation for Health Communities/New
Hampshire Partnership for End-of-Life Care)
www.healthnh.com/fhc/initiatives/performance/eol/eolreports.php

Forms: Advance Directive (Foundation for Health Communities/New
Hampshire Partnership for End-of-Life Care)
www.healthnh.com/fhc/initiatives/performance/eol/ACPG 2007
revisions.pdf

*New Jersey*

Advance Directives for Health Care (Commission on Legal and Ethical
Problems in the Delivery of Health Care)
www.state.nj.us/health/healthfacilities/documents/ltc/advance_directives
.pdf

Advance Directives in New Jersey (Ombudsman for the Institutionalized
Elderly)
www.state.nj.us/health/healthfacilities/documents/ltc/advance_directives
_brochure.pdf

Forms: Combined Advance Directive for Health Care, Instruction
Directive (Commission on Legal and Ethical Problems in the Delivery of
Health Care)
www.state.nj.us/health/healthfacilities/documents/ltc/advance_directives
.pdf

### New Mexico

Advance Health Care Directives (Aging and Long-Term Services Department)
www.nmaging.state.nm.us/PDF_files/AHCDQA.pdf

Forms: Optional Advance Health Care Directive (State Bar of New Mexico)
www.nmaging.state.nm.us/pdf_files/AHCDforms.pdf

### New York

Who Will Speak for You? (Department of Health)
www.health.state.ny.us/professionals/patients/health_care_proxy/index.htm

Planning Your Health Care in Advance (Office of the Attorney General)
www.oag.state.ny.us/bureaus/health_care/pdfs/Planning Your Health Care in Advance.REVISED.pdf

Form: Health Care Proxy (Department of Health)
www.health.state.ny.us/forms/doh-1430.pdf

Form: Living Will (New York State Bar Association)
www.nysba.org/Content/NavigationMenu/PublicResources/LivingWill HealthCareProxyForms/LivingWillEnglish.pdf

Forms: Health Care Proxy, Non-Hospital Order Not to Resuscitate (Office of the Attorney General)
www.oag.state.ny.us/bureaus/health_care/pdfs/Planning Your Health Care in Advance.REVISED.pdf

### North Carolina

Medical Care Decisions and Advance Directives (Department of Health and Human Services)
www.ncdhhs.gov/dma/medicaid/AdvanceDirectExpanded.pdf

Living Wills and Health Care Power of Attorney (North Carolina Bar Association)
www.ncbar.org/media/2592940/livingwills.pdf

End-of-Life Resources (North Carolina Medical Society)
www.ncmedsoc.org/pages/public_health_info/end_of_life.html

Advance Health Care Directive Registry (Secretary of State)
www.secretary.state.nc.us/ahcdr

Form: Health Care Power of Attorney (North Carolina Medical
Society)
www.ncmedsoc.org/non_members/public_resources/hcpowerofattorney
2007.pdf

Form: Advance Directive for a Natural Death ("Living Will") (North
Carolina Medical Society)
www.ncmedsoc.org/non_members/public_resources/livingwillform.pdf

### North Dakota

Making Health Care Decisions in North Dakota (Department of Human
Services)
www.nd.gov/dhs/info/pubs/docs/aging/aging-healthcare-directives-guide
.pdf

Form: Health Care Directive (Department of Human Services)
www.nd.gov/dhs/info/pubs/docs/aging/aging-healthcare-directives-guide
.pdf

### Ohio

Advance Directives (Ohio Legal Rights Service)
http://olrs.ohio.gov/asp/olrs_AdvanceDirect.asp

Forms: Living Will Declaration, Donor Registry Enrollment Form, Health
Care Power of Attorney (Ohio State Bar Association)
www.ohiobar.org/AdvanceDirectives/practiceaids/advancedirectives/
advance directives-09update.pdf

Form: Durable Power of Attorney for Health Care (Ohio Legal Rights
Service)
http://olrs.ohio.gov/asp/olrs_AdvanceDirect.asp

### Oklahoma

End-of-Life Health Care (Office of the Attorney General)
www.oag.state.ok.us/oagweb.nsf/AdvanceDirective

FAQs for Advance Planning (Oklahoma Palliative Care Resource Center
at the University of Oklahoma)
www.fammed.ouhsc.edu/Palliative-Care/FAQsAboutAdvanceDirectives
.htm

Advance Directive for Health Care (Living Will)—Frequently Asked
Questions (Oklahoma Bar Association)
www.okbar.org/public/brochures/advancedQA.htm

Form: Advance Directive for Health Care (Oklahoma Bar Association)
www.okbar.org/public/brochures/AdvDirective2006.pdf

### Oregon

Advance Directives (Department of Consumer and Business Services)
http://egov.oregon.gov/DCBS/SHIBA/advanced_directives.shtml

What Is a Living Will? (Oregon State Bar)
www.osbar.org/public/legalinfo/1120_LivingWill.htm

Form: Advance Directive (Department of Consumer and Business
Services)
www.oregon.gov/DCBS/SHIBA/docs/advance_directive_form.pdf

### Pennsylvania

Understanding Advance Directives for Health Care (Department of
Aging)
www.portal.state.pa.us/portal/server.pt?open=514&objID=616385
&mode=2

Advance Health Care Declaration (Living Will) (Pennsylvania Bar
Association)
www.pabar.org/clips/AdvanceHealthCareDirective.pdf

Advance Directives (Pennsylvania Medical Society)
www.pamedsoc.org/advancedirectives

Form: Durable Health Care Power of Attorney and Health Care
Treatment Instructions (Department of Aging)
www.dsf.health.state.pa.us/health/lib/health/publicnotices/Sample
_Forms_for_Advance_Directives.pdf

*Rhode Island*

End of Life Care (Office of the Attorney General)
www.riag.ri.gov/civilcriminal/endoflife.php

Forms: Durable Power of Attorney for Health Care, Living Will (Office of
the Attorney General)
www.riag.ri.gov/civilcriminal/endoflife.php

Forms: Durable Power of Attorney for Health Care, Living Will (Department of Health)
www.health.ri.gov/lifestages/death/about/livingwill/

*South Carolina*

Advance Directives (Office on Aging)
http://aging.sc.gov/legal/Pages/AdvanceDirectives.aspx

Forms: Living Will, Health Care Power of Attorney (Office on Aging)
http://aging.sc.gov/legal/Pages/LivingWillAndPowerOfAttorney.aspx

*South Dakota*

Planning for Health Care Decisions (State Bar of South Dakota)
www.sdbar.org/pamphlets/healthcare.shtm

Advance Directives (South Dakota State Medical Association)
www.sdsma.org/publichealthscience/healthscienceinit/documents/
AdvanceDirectiveFinal_000.pdf

Form: Living Will Declaration (State Bar of South Dakota)
www.sdbar.org/pamphlets/Living_Will.html

*Tennessee*

Advance Directives Resources (Department of Health)
http://health.state.tn.us/AdvanceDirectives/index.htm

Forms: Advanced Care Plan, Appointment of Health Care Agent
(Department of Health)
http://health.state.tn.us/AdvanceDirectives/index.htm

*Texas*

Legal Planning: Questions and Answers (Department of State Health
Services)
www.dshs.state.tx.us/alzheimers/legal.shtm

Medical Power of Attorney (Texas Medical Association)
www.texmed.org/Template.aspx?id=65

Forms: Directive to Physicians and Family or Surrogate, Medical
Power of Attorney, Out-of-Hospital Do Not Resuscitate Information
(Department of Aging and Disability Services)
www.dads.state.tx.us/news_info/publications/handbooks/index.html

Form: Directive to Physicians and Family or Surrogate, Medical
Power of Attorney (State Bar of Texas/Texas Young Lawyers
Association)
www.tyla.org/tasks/sites/tyla/assets/File/directive.pdf

Form: Medical Power of Attorney (State Bar of Texas/Texas Young
Lawyers Association)
www.tyla.org/tasks/sites/tyla/assets/File/medicalpoa.pdf

*Utah*

Advance Directives (Department of Human Services)
www.hsdaas.utah.gov/advance_directives.htm

Form: Advance Healthcare Directive (Department of Human Services)
www.hsdaas.utah.gov/pdf/FORM.pdf

Form: Advance Healthcare Directive (Utah State Bar)
www.utahbar.org/sections/yld/willsforheroes/assets/adv_health_care
_directive.pdf

*Vermont*

End of Life Issues (Vermont Medical Association)
www.vtmd.org/end-life-issues

Registering an Advance Directive (Department of Health)
http://healthvermont.gov/vadr/register.aspx

Form: Advance Directive for Health Care (Department of Health)
http://healthvermont.gov/regs/ad/AD_attachmentA.pdf

Form: Advance Directive Registry Registration Agreement (Department
of Health)
Form: http://healthvermont.gov/regs/ad/AD_registration_agreement.pdf

*Virginia*

Advance Medical Directive (Department for the Aging)
www.vda.virginia.gov/advmedir.asp

Virginia Advance Directives (Virginia State Bar)
www.vsb.org/site/public/healthcare-decisions-day

Form: Advance Medical Directive (Department for the Aging)
www.mhav.org/uploads/VIRGINIA_CODE_FORM_AdvMedDir.pdf

Form: Advance Medical Directive (Virginia State Bar)
www.vsb.org/docs/sections/health/VA_AdvDir-2009.pdf

*Washington*

Advance Directives Q & A (Washington State Medical Association)
www.wsma.org/patient_resources/advance-directives-qa.cfm

Legal Planning [including advance directives] (Department of Social and
Health Services, Aging and Disability Services Administration)
http://www.adsa.dshs.wa.gov/pubinfo/legal/#advance

Washington State Living Will Registry (Department of Health)
www.doh.wa.gov/livingwill

Form: Durable Power of Attorney for Health Care (Washington State Medical Association)
www.wsma.org/files/Downloads/PatientResources/HCD-forms.pdf

Forms: Health Care Directive, Durable Power of Attorney for Health Care (Department of Health)
www.doh.wa.gov/livingwill/registerdocuments.htm

### West Virginia

Advance Directives for Health Care Decision-Making in West Virginia: Frequently Asked Questions (West Virginia Center for End-of-Life Care)
www.hsc.wvu.edu/chel/wvi/_pdf/faq_2009.pdf

Information for Patients and Families (West Virginia Center for End-of-Life Care)
www.hsc.wvu.edu/chel/wvi/patient_family_home.html

Forms: Living Will, Medical Power of Attorney, Combined Living Will & Medical Power of Attorney (West Virginia Center for End-of-Life Care)
www.hsc.wvu.edu/chel/wvi/_pdf/faq_2009.pdf

### Wisconsin

Your Right to Direct Your Future Health Needs (Department of Health Services)
http://dhs.wisconsin.gov/bqaconsumer/NursingHomes/NHneeds.htm

Advance Directives (State Bar of Wisconsin)
www.wisbar.org/AM/Template.cfm?Section=LifePlanning&Template=/CM/ContentDisplay.cfm&ContentID=38080

Forms: Declaration to Physicians (Living Will), Power of Attorney for Health Care (Department of Health Services)
http://dhs.wisconsin.gov/forms/AdvDirectives/ADFormsPOA.htm

Form: Living Will (State Bar of Wisconsin)
www.wisbar.org/AM/Template.cfm?Section=LifePlanning&Template=/
CM/ContentDisplay.cfm&ContentID=38085

Form: Power of Attorney for Health Care (State Bar of Wisconsin)
www.wisbar.org/AM/Template.cfm?Section=LifePlanning&Template=/
CM/ContentDisplay.cfm&ContentID=38086

### Wyoming

Comfort One Program (Wyoming Department of Health)
http://wdh.state.wy.us/sho/comfortone/index.html

Information Concerning the Durable Power of Attorney for Health Care
(Wyoming State Bar)
https://www.wyomingbar.org/pdf/forms/Info_Durable_Power_of
_Attorney.pdf

Form: Advance Health Care Directive (Department of Health/Wyoming
AARP)
http://health.wyo.gov/Media.aspx?mediaId=2699

# Index

.........................................................................................

death (*continued*)
at home, 17, 25, 53, 94, 95, 117;
modern estrangement from, 10;
natural, 17, 56; and Quinlan
case, 65–66; right to, 65–66,
67–68, 69; and Schiavo, 69; and
self-determination, 4. *See also*
dying; end of life
death panels, 20, 109
dementia, 30, 31, 32, 99, 100, 101–2.
*See also* Alzheimer's disease
depression, 21, 85, 97
diazepam (Valium), 23
Dilaudid, 59
Donate Life organization, 75–76
dronabinol (Marinol), 23
Drug Enforcement Agency (DEA),
22, 23
dying: contemplation of, 16; fear
of, 12, 87; and hospice, 85, 87;
modern estrangement from, 10;
and self-determination, 4. *See also*
death; end of life

Eckhart, Dave, 71–77, 81
electroencephalogram (EEG), 58
embolism, 49, 50, 72
end of life: concerns about care at,
12, 109; economics of care at,
25–26; expenses at, 121; and
hospice, 85, 86; and palliative care,
84; participation in decisions
about, 4–5. *See also* death; dying
epinephrine, 60
estate planning, 10, 110. *See also*
inheritance
euthanasia, 64. *See also* assisted
suicide

family: and Bill Johnson, 3; burden
to, 119; and Cole, 30–31, 34–35,
36; copy of advance directive for,
43, 114; disagreements among, 5,
34–35, 79, 81, 121; and Eckhart,
74–76, 81; and experience of
dying, 25; and hospice, 86, 87;

isolation from, 3; and Harold
Johnson, 1, 2; and Kranz, 52; and
Miller, 89, 90, 91, 92, 93, 94, 96;
and palliative care, 83; and patient's
preferences, 54; and Quinlan case,
65; and Schiavo case, 69; and
Simmons, 45–46, 47–49
Federal District Court, 70
fentanyl, 20
Five Wishes, 42
Five Wishes party, 110
friends, 2, 3, 16, 43, 48, 96, 97, 119
funerals, 28, 41, 95, 96–97, 117–18

guardian, 64, 65, 66, 67–68, 69

Hawking, Stephen, 48
health care: decisions about, 42;
instructions for, 27, 41, 55–61;
personal cost of, 35
health care agent, 43, 52, 75, 90,
103–4, 113, 114, 120; selection
of, 27, 41, 55, 79–81
health care costs, 25–26, 39, 80, 100,
101–2, 121
health care providers, 113, 114. *See
also* physicians
health care system, 5–6, 20, 109
heart, 1, 4, 15, 17, 66; and cardiac
arrest, 11, 31, 39, 60–61, 69
heroin, 20, 22, 23
hospice, 25, 49, 51, 83, 84, 95, 96,
114; characteristics of, 49, 85–87
hospitals, 3, 29–30, 31, 37, 38,
64–66, 80, 114; costs of, 35, 39;
death in, 25; and hospice, 86; and
insurance companies, 34; and
utilization review (UR), 34
hydration, 57–59, 67. *See also*
nutrition
hydrocodone/acetaminophen
(Lortab), 23
hydromorphone (Dilaudid), 20

incapacity, 43, 69
incompetence, 64, 65, 66, 81, 93